Extraordinary Healers

CURE Readers Honor Oncology Nurses

Volume 8

Extraordinary Healers

CURE Readers Honor Oncology Nurses

Volume 8

curemedia**group**

Plainsboro, New Jersey

Made possible with financial support from

Amgen, Inc.

Millennium: The Takeda Oncology Company

Published by
CURE Media Group
666 Plainsboro Road, Suite 300
Plainsboro, NJ 08536

Information presented is not intended as a substitute for the personalized professional advice given by a healthcare provider. This publication was produced by CURE Media Group. The views expressed in this publication are not necessarily those of the publisher. Although great care has been taken to ensure accuracy, CURE Media Group and its servants or agents shall not be responsible or in any way liable for the continued currency of the information or for any errors, omissions or inaccuracies in this book, whether arising from negligence or otherwise, or for any consequences arising therefrom. The intention of this book is not to provide specific medical advice. Essays have also been edited for grammar, style, length and clarity. Review and creation of content is solely the responsibility of CURE Media Group.

Any mention of retail products does not constitute an endorsement by the authors or the publisher.

Library of Congress Control Number: 2015937076

ISBN 978-0-692-41251-0

Introduction and interviews by Kathy LaTour
Edited by Elizabeth Whittington
Design and layout by Misty Crawford
Photo coordination by Emily Hakkinen

Printed in the United States of America

This book is dedicated to all oncology nurses who bring hope and healing to patients with cancer and their loved ones.

If you would like to give this book as a gift to your Extraordinary Healer, we've provided this page for your message.

This book honors:

_____

_____

_____

_____

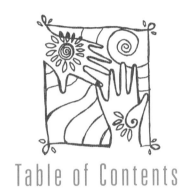

Table of Contents

Table of Contents

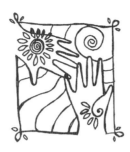

Oncology Nurses:
Giving of Their Hearts and Souls

When we began the Extraordinary Healer™ Award for Oncology Nursing eight years ago, we received essays like the ones in this book. Each essayist talked about the oncology nurse who had come into his or her life with the diagnosis of cancer, nurses who appeared at different times in their journey to care for them in ways above and beyond their job description.

Having been there, I could identify with the essayists who found a voice, a touch or a look that told them they were not alone.

Each year the staff of *CURE* decided which essays best exemplified the spirit of the extraordinary healer, often after hours of debate and what can only be called passionate discussion. How do you choose between a nurse who fills out hours of paperwork to get "compassionate use" for a drug not yet available and the nurse who makes it possible for her patient to go to the prom without her infusion backpack by going to her house to remove it before she leaves and then returning to reattach it at 4 a.m. when the young patient returns home.

I can remember thinking there was no way we would hear such stories the second year or the third or the fourth or the fifth. And yet they came. The nurse who made two five-hour drives with her patient to the large cancer center where she could learn how to administer the chemotherapy they had designed so her patient could be at home for her treatments. Or the nurse who took early retirement from a major corporation because he felt called to be an oncology nurse. Then there was the oncology nurse who drove through 16 inches of snow to deliver a packet of information needed for the patient to understand her options–on Christmas Eve before the roads were plowed.

One 17-year old who had battled cancer since age 6 wrote in his essay about his nurse and her ability to

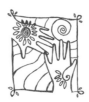

always make his days in the hospital special. On his birthday he was feeling alone when the door opened to friends, balloons and his nurse, who was there on her day off not only to take part, but to sing him a song she had written for him. We heard about birthdays, special events and even a wedding planned by the oncology nurse of a young man whose fiancé knew they would never leave the hospital.

Every year we read them and cried. How do people give so much over and over?

I think I finally read the answer in one essay that has stayed with me. The mother about her daughter, who was diagnosed with a rare cancer the week after she graduated from college.

Her descriptions took me to this young woman's life where I could actually see this chemotherapy nurse as she cared for her daughter with laughter, patience and love. The mother wrote of how the nurse orchestrated her daughter's magic night with Justin Timberlake, her request from the Make-a-Wish Foundation. She recounted all the times their special nurse was present, for the good, the bad, the ugly—and the end.

It was Good Friday morning, and the nurse left her oncology station to drive to the hospice where the young woman was spending her final days. Not having seen her since chemotherapy ended, she later told her mother that she didn't know what drew her to her daughter's bedside that day except that she knew somehow the time was short. And it was. Her family had decided a drug-induced coma would begin within hours of the nurse's arrival. It was her last opportunity to say goodbye, which she did, grasping the young woman and pulling her to her chest, and, as her mother saw, "into her heart."

Then I remembered how in judging the essays, we had become so weary of every essayist calling their nurse an angel.

We were wrong. They are angels, every one of them.

—Kathy LaTour

Extraordinary Healers

Our Winner
& Finalists

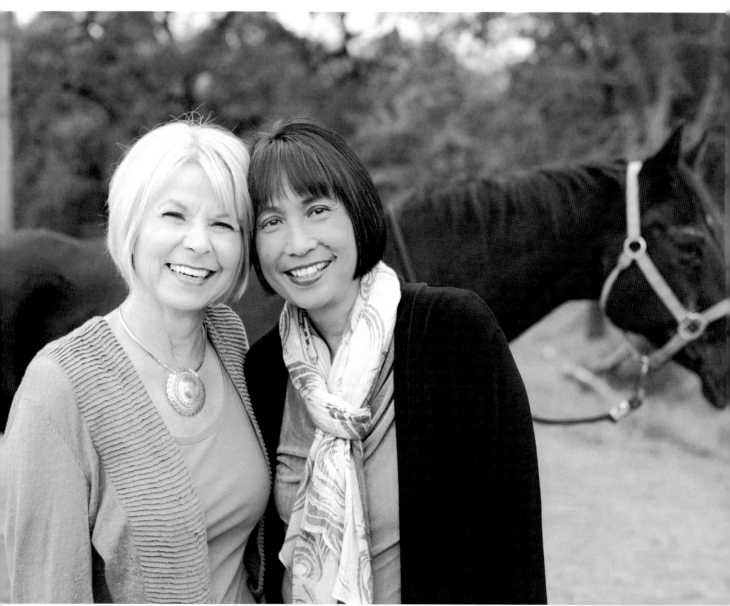

Cynthia Cantril, RN, OCN, MPH, with Ann Tallman [right]

The Gift of Giving

WINNER OF THE 2014 EXTRAORDINARY HEALER AWARD FOR ONCOLOGY NURSING

CYNTHIA "CINDI" CANTRIL, RN, OCN, MPH

[SUTTER PACIFIC MEDICAL FOUNDATION IN SANTA ROSA, CALIFORNIA]

WRITTEN BY ANN TALLMAN

IT'S NOT EVERY DAY that one receives a cancer diagnosis. I've been healthy all my life. Cancer doesn't happen to me; it happens to "them." Then I discovered that it can happen to anyone—it happened to me. The two words that every woman fears: breast cancer.

I DIDN'T realize that my whole life was about to change. That was when I first met Cindi Cantril. She had the unpleasant task of giving me the news. I knew when we first met that she was someone I could trust. Little did I know that she would become a huge part of my life.

It wasn't what she said or did. It was the feeling of compassion and sincerity with which she spoke. It was the confidence and reassurance in her voice that she'd walk with me every step of the way and that I'd get through treatment.

It's her dedication to serve, her desire to give unselfishly of herself, her commitment to helping women. And she does it all with a great smile and a positive attitude.

Cindi is one of those special people who was blessed with the gift of serving, of giving unconditionally from the heart.

Once I received my diagnosis, she and her team at Cancer Support Services and Patient Navigation banded together and assisted me every step of the way, scheduling tests and physician referrals, advising me on what to expect and providing information to help me make good, sound decisions on my treatment options. She became a member of our family, supporting my husband and our children.

The big day was upon us: surgery. As I sat with my husband, Jerry, in the waiting room for my presurgical wire implant, I began to feel a lot of anxiety building up. Cindi had shared some relaxation exercises with me, and I just couldn't get myself to settle down, even with Jerry by my side.

Out of the blue, I felt someone sit beside me and take a hold of my hand. I looked up, and there was Cindi, smiling and reassuring me that everything would be all right.

She met me in the room where the procedure was about to take place. She made sure I was comfortable and relaxed, and then she left the room. Unbeknownst to me, she went out to the waiting room to be with Jerry, providing support and a shoulder to lean on.

It isn't that she's done one thing that's really extraordinary—it's the extraordinary things she does every day.

All of this started in November 2010, and she is still a part of our lives today. In her ongoing quest to serve women, Cindi was the backbone in the development of our peer-to-peer support program called WINGS—Women Inspiring, Nurturing, Giving, Supporting.

The development of WINGS came about when Cindi saw a need for a program where women could help other women with a similar diagnosis. She looked at existing programs across the country as models for the program she intended to develop. She took the best practices from several established programs and put together a program that would work for our community. Once the framework was set, she hand selected the first group of volunteers.

Working tirelessly, the volunteers (I happen to be one of them) were trained to listen generously with an open ear and an open heart. Many newly diagnosed women have been paired up with volunteers, and the results have been amazing. The program has been so successful that it's expanded to support not only breast cancer patients, but women with other types of cancers and a men's group—WINGMEN.

Cindi has done numerous presentations on WINGS and is working diligently to expand the program to other facilities.

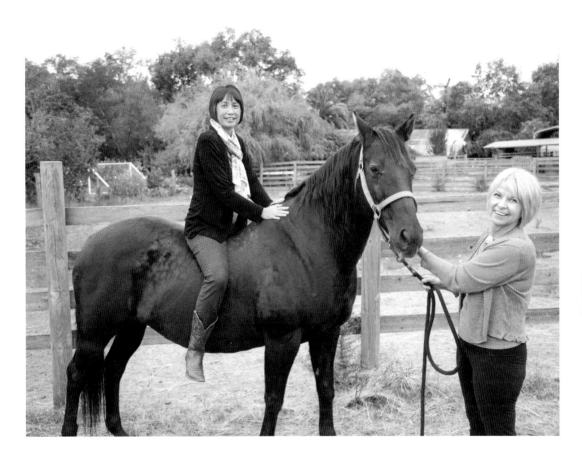

Outside the office, Cindi is an avid equestrian at heart. She's combined her love of horses with her desire to help patients heal by developing Sutter Cancer Support Services' equine facilitated therapy program.

Cancer treatment is more than diagnosis, surgery, radiation and chemotherapy. It is also a healing of the mind, body and spirit. The healing power of horses cannot be explained, not by science anyway.

I learned about the principles of horsemanship, about reconnecting to the natural world. I learned to focus on the here and now, not the maybe's and what if's. It renewed a lot of values that had somehow gotten lost in this busy world, values such as trust, respect and partnership. I learned to trust my intuition rather than to question it. And I've learned to become more curious about the world around me, curious about what I can do to make it a better place.

On the clinical side, participants had salivary swabs taken three times a day during the program that were used to measure salivary cortisol levels in the morning, before working with the horses and after. As expected, cortisol levels dropped measurably over the course of the program.

Yes, science was very instrumental in measuring cortisol levels; however, we have yet to find out why these changes occurred.

Cancer treatment is stressful, and Cindi understands how much it takes out of a patient. In an effort to help women heal even more, she organizes annual three-day retreats for cancer patients, so they can pamper themselves, meditate, share their experiences and help one another heal. She brings together an amazing group of speakers and coordinates activities that energize the spirit.

Cindi has been a member of our community in Santa Rosa, California, since 2010 and has brought all of these programs to reality. That's quite an amazing feat for such a short amount of time.

The lives she has touched and the impact she's had on so many women and their families cannot be measured. Cancer, believe it or not, has changed my life for the better, and I would never have met this remarkable woman otherwise. It isn't that she's done one thing that's really extraordinary—it's the extraordinary things she does every day. ❧

On the Wings of Angels

AN INTERVIEW WITH CINDI CANTRIL, RN, OCN, MPH

CINDI CANTRIL, RN, OCN, MPH, remembers only the eyes of her patients. She was 15 and volunteering with patients who had head and neck cancer while her mother was finishing her nursing degree. Their heads had been bandaged completely after surgery, so they couldn't speak. Only their eyes told her what they needed. It was the moment that she says she knew she wanted to speak for cancer patients.

SHE ENTERED nursing school as soon as she graduated from high school, beginning her advocacy then and continuing it today as the Clinical Breast Care Nurse for Sutter Health in Santa Rosa, California. She is also the 2014 recipient of CURE's Extraordinary Healer Award for Oncology Nursing.

"My mother finished nursing school at 51, and I worked at the hospital as a volunteer when I was a teenager; my very first support group had patients with cancer on the roof of their mouth, melanoma, thyroid cancer, ovarian cancer."

Cindi didn't care. It was a sacred space to her patients and to her, a place where people were heard.

Today, Cindi meets breast cancer patients and sets them up for biopsies. She is also the one who tells them they have breast cancer.

"I know the words I say are going to change her life," she says. "I tell them what I think the next six months will look like and then focus on now."

She is grateful that she meets them before the diagnosis because it gives her a chance to see who they are and gauge how well they will take the news.

"It's a dance because I have to read them. Before the biopsy I can determine how well she will handle it when I tell her."

As part of her work, she has established a monthly support group called WINGS—Women Inspiring, Nurturing, Giving, Supporting, where women can gather to talk about where they are and how they are. Trained volunteers work one-on-one with the patients and are available for calls and with their time. She also began an equestrian program for the patients.

"We had breast cancer survivors come to the barn for an hour for two weeks. They said cancer was so big that when they felt confident around a 1,200-pound animal, they felt more in control of the cancer," she says.

It's the size, she adds, that helps patients learn to be in the present and not think about chemotherapy. Instead, they are aware of the massive animal nuzzling their arm. Cindi and her staff train volunteers on an ongoing basis and then, because they know them, they can match them with newly diagnosed patients.

Cindi is not modest when it comes to understanding that she has a gift. Rather, she understands it is her job to recognize her gift, nurture it and respect it—and use it with her patients to guide them through the breast cancer journey. ❧

TEACHING MOMENT:

"I know the words I say are going to change her life," she says. "I tell them what I think the next six months will look like and then focus on now."

My Dad's Dime

NOELLE PAUL, RN, BSN, OCN, CAPA [MEMORIAL SLOAN KETTERING CANCER CENTER IN NEW YORK, NEW YORK]

WRITTEN BY MARY KAY MORELLI

MY FATHER PASSED AWAY very suddenly in October 2007. Ever since I was a little girl, my dad and I had a special thing about dimes. I always loved the sound of jingling change in his pants pocket. We would play a game, and I remember his laughter as I would always take the bigger coins from his pocket, leaving him with just the dimes because they were the smallest. Ever since he passed, I find dimes in random places, especially when I really need a hug, some advice or, more recently, strength.

OUR CANCER story began on a perfect August night. We went as a family to watch our son Jack play football. My husband, Mike, was running around with the kids during warm-up and you could just see him having a great time being their coach. The next morning, I received a call from Mike telling me that his back was hurting. I knew something was wrong when I suggested he go to the ER and he agreed. They ran numerous tests, including a CT scan and blood work, and within hours he was admitted. The love of my life had received a diagnosis of colorectal cancer at age 40.

The next few days seemed like a blur as we went from the shock of hearing this diagnosis to a full on press on how we beat it. In the blink of an eye, our lives were turned upside down, or, as I like to say, turned on a dime. This story is about finding our real life dime that gives us strength as we fight this battle against cancer together.

Her name is Noelle Paul. She is a nurse at Memorial Sloan Kettering Cancer Center in New York City.

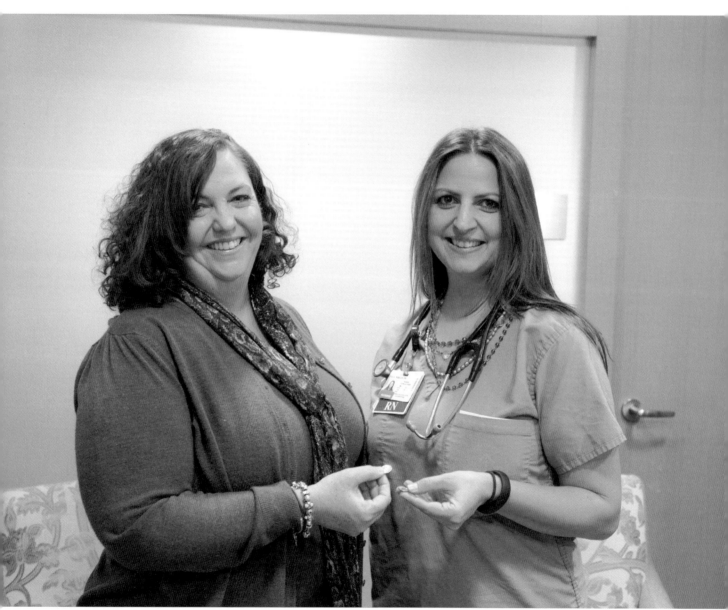

Mary Kay Morelli, with Noelle Paul, RN, BSN, OCN, CAPA, [right]

We first met Noelle on June 14, 2012, at the first of what would be many surgeries for my husband's cancer. She walked into the waiting room and called his name. As we stood up to meet her, she bent down to hand me a dime that I had dropped out of my pocket. Little did I know, but that was my dad's way of telling me to be strong and not to worry. He had sent me Noelle. It would take me a year and about 30 surgeries with her as my husband's nurse to fully understand the power of my dad's dime that day.

Noelle has been responsible for Mike's care on over 30 separate surgeries. When we would discover that Noelle had been assigned as his nurse, our level of anxiety about the pending procedure would immediately decrease. We knew that she was incredibly knowledgeable and always on top of her game. It made having the surgeries much easier for the both of us.

She was always aware of any new developments or side effects my husband was experiencing with his chemotherapy. As my husband's health changed, Noelle maintained excellent communication with the surgeons, surgical nursing staff and anesthesia team. She made sure everyone involved in his care stayed informed of his health conditions. She was committed to giving my husband the best care possible, and is, by far, the most intelligent nurse we have ever come into contact with. And we have met a lot of nurses on this journey.

During these surgeries, we got to know each other pretty well. Although Noelle always remained vigilant and took her job very seriously, she would find time to ask about our three young kids.

Her compassion toward

TEACHING MOMENT:

As my husband's health changed, Noelle maintained excellent communication with the surgeons, surgical nursing staff and anesthesia team. She made sure everyone involved in his care stayed informed of his health conditions.

me as a caregiver has to be my favorite thing about her. On June 19, 2013, my husband endured a major surgery that lasted more than 22 hours. Noelle changed her schedule to make sure she was working that day to take care of Mike prior to surgery. Her dedication did not end there. After completing her 12-hour shift that day, instead of going home, Noelle stayed by my side, comforting me for another 14 hours. She kept me strong for my husband as he was transferred from surgery to the ICU.

Sitting in the waiting room with Noelle, I finally shared with her my story about my dad and the dime. By the end of the story, we were both in tears. Initially, I wasn't quite sure why she was crying, but out of her pocket, she pulled a dime. She explained to me that she had found it that morning. As the goose bumps on my arm made their way to the back of my neck, I pulled out the dime I had found at breakfast that morning. It was at that moment that I knew where my strength was coming from—it was from my guardian angel, Noelle, who just so happens to be the most dedicated cancer nurse we have ever met.

Without Noelle, I am not sure how we would have made it. Most people only have a few surgeries during their cancer battle. We, unfortunately, had more than what is considered normal. Without Noelle as part of our team, we would not have had the strength to continue. I still find dimes from my dad, but I smile and know that he sent us more than a dime; he sent us a nurse who is truly an extraordinary healer. Noelle Paul is simply the best! ❧

Making a Difference

AN INTERVIEW WITH NOELLE PAUL, RN, BSN, OCN, CAPA

NOELLE PAUL, RN, BSN, OCN, CAPA, has time to talk on the way home from her job as an oncology surgical nurse at Memorial Sloan Kettering Cancer Center in New York City. Today, she only stayed an hour past her shift, but she explains that she needed to spend time with a patient whose surgery was postponed until tomorrow.

"SHE WAS so nervous anyway. I needed to keep her distracted and calm until there was someone who could spend some time with her. Being there with her and keeping her distracted was so important."

Paul decided to become a nurse in high school. "I loved science and wanted to do something in health care. I could see what a different relationship patients had with nurses than with doctors."

Oncology nursing came about when she cared for a patient during an internship in nursing school. As it is with many oncology nurses, she went where they needed her and then never left. "I found an affinity with the cancer patients. They were complex and there was a psychosocial side."

She recalls the patient with head and neck cancer in his 30s and how very hard it was for him after a devastating surgery.

"I took care of him from pre-surgery to when he went home. His family was devastated. I got to make a real difference in his life and got to know his family and be involved."

For Paul, it's about making a difference no matter the outcome for patients experiencing the most dramatic moments of their lives.

After 15 years of oncology nursing at Sloan Kettering, she says her decision has been affirmed many times by her patients as she prepares them for surgery and then stays with them afterward.

———

"We have also seen so many advances in the diagnosis that used to be a death sentence. The quality and quantity of life have changed for cancer patients."

Paul says she is grateful to be a nurse in oncology and for what she has learned from her patients about perseverance and strength and an unwillingness to give up—even when the patients die, she says.

"We can be present to be sure they are getting the things that contribute to a peaceful end." ❧

TEACHING MOMENT:

Paul says she is grateful to be a nurse in oncology and for what she has learned from her patients about perseverance and strength and an unwillingness to give up—even when the patients die, she says.

If You Need Me,
Call and I Will Be There

ANNE TODD, RN, OCN [SOUTHERN INDIANA PHYSICIANS IU HEALTH ONCOLOGY IN BLOOMINGTON, INDIANA]

WRITTEN BY CHUCK WILSON

THE JOURNEY has been long and hard, and the light at the end of the tunnel appears to be an oncoming train instead of a ray of hope. After many visits, to many states, to see many aides, nurses, assistants and doctors, Ann Todd, of Southern Indiana Physicians IU Health Oncology, has managed to show us what patient care is all about. And that oncoming train has miraculously left the tracks.

Winner & Finalists

IT ALL began with a CT scan to check the esophagus. There is no way we could have expected or been prepared for the results … esophageal cancer at the GE junction. Upon further examination, the cancer had spread to the liver, as well. Being stage 4, we knew the odds were not in our favor and there was no real cure.

It is amazing how quickly your life turns upside down when you receive news of cancer. And, you are not the only one affected. Your family members, friends, loved ones, work colleagues and the list goes on.

There are so many good oncology teams in this country treating cancer, and it is difficult assessing the abilities of the caregivers knowing that there can never be an apples-to-apples comparison based on the needs and differences of each and every patient. We have traveled the Midwest seeking care, so we have experienced many differences in patient care.

Many years ago, my golden retriever was very ill, so I carried him to my vehicle and took him to the vet. Upon arrival, the doctor came to the back of my vehicle, crawled in, held him and cried. I tell you this story because that is the standard that I set in all care. The bar can never be set high enough when it comes to patient care. There have been many who have come close; however, Anne Todd has reached that level of care and concern for her patients.

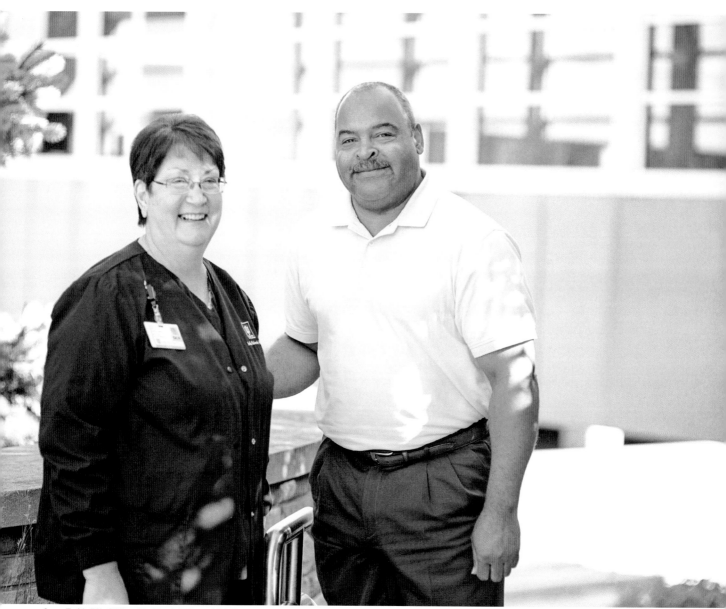

Anne Todd, RN, OCN, with Chuck Wilson [right]

Anne has given professionalism a new meaning. Yes, it is one thing to be professional; however, it is something completely different when professionalism is blended with compassion, care, empathy, concern, understanding and overall awareness of the needs of those she is serving. A good meal can be quickly ruined by poor service, just as with patient care.

Outside of the appointments, Anne calls on a regular basis to make sure everything is OK and ask if there is anything she could do to make the family more comfortable. Anne made arrangements with her church to help supply needed funds to purchase nutrition since the insurance company did not cover this expense. Anne also pulled together a few of her friends and came over to help clean the home, do laundry, and though she claims not to know what to cook, she offered to prepare food as well.

The thing that stands out most in my mind is what Anne did outside the office. Anne, with a few others, made arrangements to send the family to Disney World over the Christmas holiday. With medical bills, medications and other expenses, there is no money for things like trips or even Christmas gifts. Anne and her friends made sure there was a Christmas for the family. Nothing was left undone. Transportation, lodging, money, medication and nutrition were all arranged so the family could enjoy this precious time together. Anne and those involved were not part of the rich and famous (though they deserve to be). They gave up time-shares, frequent flier miles and took up a collection to make sure the family wanted

TEACHING MOMENT:

It is one thing to be professional; however, it is something completely different when professionalism is blended with compassion, care, empathy, concern, understanding and overall awareness of the needs of those she is serving.

for nothing during this trip.

I was taught the best thing you can do for another is to give of yourself, and that is why I truly believe Anne Todd has risen to that standard. Anne gave of herself to one she only recently met. She pulled together resources that seemed impossible to create a memory for those left behind to cherish for a lifetime.

I will close by reciting a quote by Julian of Norwich: "A cheerful giver does not count the cost of what he gives. His heart is set on pleasing and cheering him to whom the gift is given." Anne has earned my respect, trust and admiration. ✼

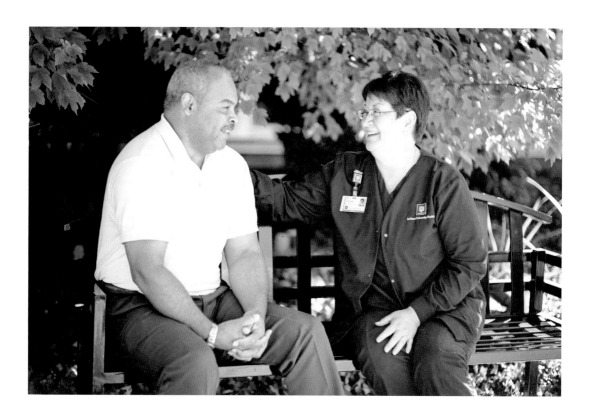

A Certain Kind of Nurse

AN INTERVIEW WITH ANNE TODD, RN, OCN

FOR 19 YEARS, Anne Todd served as a secretary in an oncology office where the doctor enjoyed teaching her about the disease.

"HE WOULD SAY, 'Anne, come and see.' He really enjoyed teaching me about oncology."

His encouragement and teaching led Todd to deciding to return to college to earn her nursing degree—at the same time her two oldest daughters were in college. She already had an affinity for patients dealing with cancer, so it wasn't a surprise when she choose oncology as her field of interest.

She knows it's not for everyone and has seen many young nurses choose another direction. Indeed, one of her first managers told new oncology nurses that if they couldn't handle oncology, she would find them another area, an offer that Todd says is not often made by nurse managers. She understood that oncology nurses have to be a certain kind of nurse.

After working in the hospital for a number of years, she is now the nurse for two oncologists at Southern Indiana Physicians Hematology Oncology in a rural area of nine counties. They laugh at the fact that she knows most of the people who walk through the doors—and is related to the rest of them. The rural factor also plays out for new nurses who have to care for older men who have worked in rock quarries and stone mills, and who may have trouble with nurses.

"I had an IU nursing student, and she came to me when an older gentleman would not let her do her assessment."

Todd walked in and started talking to him about his last name and who he was related to and working at the stone mill. By the time she was finished chatting, the young nurse had all the details for her assessment. "I told her that older men want to talk about their jobs and what they accomplished, so she needs to do that to create rapport."

Connecting with her patients is what Todd finds the most satisfying about her job. She spends numerous hours on the phone helping them with chemotherapy side effects, and on the few occasions when she has to consult with the doctor, she calls before the end of day so they don't have to wait and wonder.

"A few weeks ago I was in the exam room when the doctor told a patient the cancer was completely gone," she says, clearly choking up. "We get to celebrate the good outcomes and hold the hands of those who have bad outcomes to support them."

The previous week, Todd says, they lost two patients who had been with them since the practice opened in 2013. When patients such as these come in, Todd says she puts her phone on voice mail and spends some time with them.

The greatest compliment comes from patients, Todd says.

"I was in the grocery store last week, and one of my former patients ran into me. She said, 'You are my favorite nurse!'" ✤

CHAPTER 1
Above & Beyond

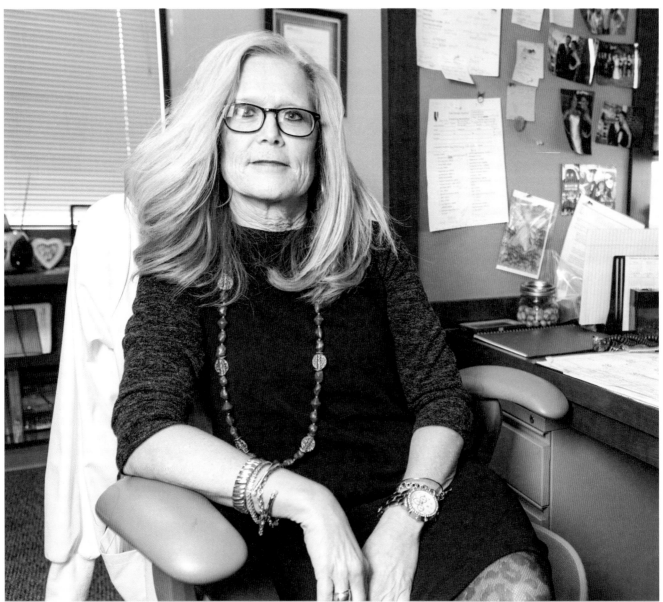

Teri Tasler, RN, OCN, CN-4

A Thousand Words Are Not Enough

TERI TASLER, RN, OCN, CN-4 [DUKE RALEIGH CANCER CENTER IN RALEIGH, NORTH CAROLINA]

WRITTEN BY CINDY BRISSON

HAVING THE DIAGNOSIS of cancer is unexplainable, and until you've been told those words, you could never imagine. Even though I'm extremely grateful for every day I wake up, living with cancer is still difficult. I have been in and out of chemotherapy and radiation for the past seven years, and my nurse Teri has always been by my side, making things a little less scary and a whole lot easier.

Above & Beyond

TERI TASLER, RN, has been my nurse for the past seven years. During those seven years, she has stayed late, arrived early, held my hand, gave me hugs, provided support, given words of encouragement and made thousands of phone calls and faxes, and probably just as many emails, all for me. In addition, she has demonstrated exceptional nursing skills. I have no idea how many patients she has, but I know it's a lot. I also know I'm not the only one; however, she always makes me feel that I'm the only one.

I was in treatment, receiving three different chemotherapy drugs and struggling with the side effects: nausea, fatigue, low blood counts and low platelets. My family had planned a trip to San Francisco for a couple of weeks. My family didn't think I would be able to go, but with Teri's help, I was on the plane with the rest of them.

Teri made calls and sent emails and faxes for days trying to make arrangements for me. At the time, I had to get blood transfusions every couple of weeks. Teri made contact with a physician in San Francisco who agreed to see me while I was there and check my blood counts and stay in touch with my doctor here in North Carolina.

Before I left, I had an appointment with an oncologist for blood work and a follow-up once a week while

I was in California. During my vacation, I ended up with a low platelet count and required an infusion of platelets. It was at night, but I was able to call Teri and she talked with the physician regarding my diagnosis of cancer and history of low platelets and low blood, which made things go much easier. She also called me the next day to check on me. The next week, when I had blood work drawn, she made sure she got the results from California and forwarded them to my doctor here in North Carolina. I was able to enjoy the trip knowing Teri would be right there on the phone, making sure I was taken care of.

As an artist, one of my dreams has always been to go to the Louvre Museum. My family planned a trip to make that happen. Even though I wasn't currently in treatment, I was still having frequent blood work and dealing with side effects from the latest chemo and radiation.

Teri worked with the physicians and made sure I had plenty of fluids and that all my counts and levels were up to par before taking the trip. Two weeks before the trip, during a follow-up scan after radiation, the physicians discovered a blood clot in my inferior vena cava. I was put on injections twice daily for the clot.

On the way home from the scan, I called Teri and told her about the clot and my hesitation about the injections. Teri's words were: "Go to the pharmacy, pick up the syringes and come to my office. I'll stay here until you get here." Now that doesn't sound like a big deal, but it was already after 5 p.m., and I don't know too many nurses that will tell you they will wait on you as long as it takes for you to get there. I finally arrived at her office about an hour or so later. Teri sat down with me, talked about the shots and showed me how to give myself the injection. She made me feel as though I was her only concern and she had all the time in the world for me.

I went on the trip and had a great time, all the while knowing that if I had any questions or concerns, I

TEACHING MOMENT:

I went on the trip and had a great time, all the while knowing that if I had any questions or concerns, I could always call Teri and she would have the answer.

could always call Teri and she would have the answer.

I've called her in the middle of the day and complained of pain or an unfamiliar symptom and she has gotten me in to see the doctor that same day, telling me, "Come on over, and we'll get you in to see the doc."

Waiting on the results of a scan can be almost torturous at times. When I have scans, I never have to wait very long to find out the results. Teri calls me the same day as soon as the results are in and goes over the scan, answering any questions and easing any concerns.

Just recently, I emailed Teri on a Wednesday afternoon, complaining of pain and telling her that I needed my PCN exchanged. A couple hours later, I had an appointment scheduled for the next morning.

Teri also started a support group for gynecological cancers and attends those meetings monthly, providing support, education and friendship.

Teri is extremely attentive and observant and can tell by my voice on the phone if I'm feeling well or not.

Teri's nursing skills are exceptional, and she goes above and beyond every day. There are no words that can explain the care and support she gives. Her kindness and love show through her dedication and work every day. While not asking or expecting anything in return, she always gives 100 percent, is always there with a smile, hug, words of encouragement or anything else her patients need. While some of the things she does can seem insignificant, it's the little things she does, day in and day out, that make her stand out above the rest and make me proud to call her "my nurse." ❧

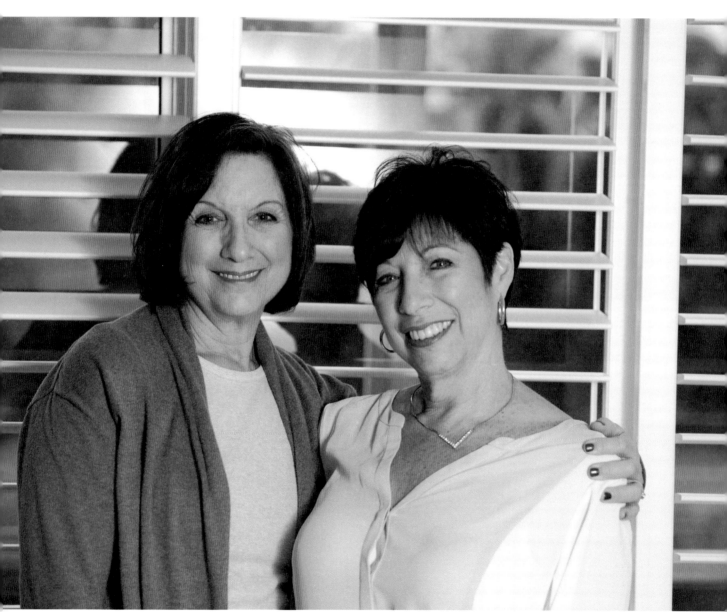

Iva Morris, RN, MSN, OCN, CNL, with Ilene Tramantano [right]

Our Mother Would Have Been So Proud

IVA MORRIS, MSN, RN, OCN, CNL

[CHARLES GEORGE VA MEDICAL CENTER IN ASHEVILLE, NORTH CAROLINA]

WRITTEN BY ILENE TRAMANTANO

I'VE ALWAYS HEARD of breast cancer survivors, but I never imagined I would become one. Not because I've never heard of women beating it, but because I've watched my own mom be diagnosed with breast cancer, and then I watched her battle it, and then I watched her lose. Now here I was, faced with my own mortality, and it was only a few years after I had witnessed my mother die before my eyes.

I HAD JUST CELEBRATED my 50th birthday, I had dreams and goals, and everything in my life was coming together according to plan. Little did I know that the universe had some other plans for me, and I would be ringing in the year with breast surgeries, chemotherapy and radiation. Like my mother, I had been diagnosed with breast cancer. I was divorced, both of my parents were now gone, my daughter had just started college. If there were ever a time where I felt the most alone, it was then.

The journey started off very routine: tests, scans and doctor appointments, and then the intensity picked up. My first surgery was flawless, so when my doctors informed me I needed a second surgery to remove my lymph nodes, I braced myself for a second go at it. When I awoke from surgery, the pain was radiating. I couldn't believe that this was happening; I wanted to die. There was no one around, and I couldn't believe I didn't see this coming.

At that moment, something changed, and in walked Nurse Iva. She headed straight for me, and instantly I felt safe and secure. She pressed the palm of my hand in hers, and I could feel the strength transferring. Just with this nurse sitting by my side, I felt everything was going to be OK.

Above & Beyond

I was discharged, and as the days went on, I felt weaker. Chemo had its grip on every breath I took. There were some days that I felt defeated. I would look at myself in the mirror and couldn't help but be reminded of my mother.

Nurse Iva started coming to my house, and it always seemed like perfect timing. Just when I thought I was out of strength, she would be there. Nurse Iva did all the things that I couldn't do for myself. She cleaned my wounds, ran the clots out of my drain, cooked for me and made sure my medicine was ready for the next day.

The worst part of being sick was I had to force my poisoned body to get up every morning, clear the fog and confusion from my head and go to work. Without me working, my daughter would never be able to finish college, and I knew it. Words cannot describe the exhaustion my body was swimming in. The only thing I can say is, those days that Nurse Iva would be at my home waiting for me after work— that kept me going. I lived for those days, because it was one of the only things that I had to look forward to.

Just with this nurse sitting by my side, I felt everything was going to be OK.

In the beginning, I would come home and crash in my clothes, in the closest spot I could find, but then Nurse Iva got me a chair for my shower. Now when I got home from work, I would let the hot water stream down my back. Sometimes I would try to slow down my thoughts, and sometimes I would cry, but that time in the shower is what Nurse Iva made me do, and I knew it was to cleanse the mind. After my showers, I would collapse on my bed, and Nurse Iva would be there to wrap me with a towel, fresh from the dryer. It was a blanket of warmth wrapping my soul. She would make me a cup of tea and lay out my clothes for the next day. When I felt I could no longer go on, Nurse Iva would look at me and remind me, "Yes, you will. You are not your mother." And I wasn't.

I have been in remission for the past 10 years. I am forever grateful to the nurse who walked with me every step of the way, through the darkest days of my life. You see, Nurse Iva is more than just an extraordinary oncology nurse to me. Nurse Iva is my sister. Our mother would have been so proud. ✿

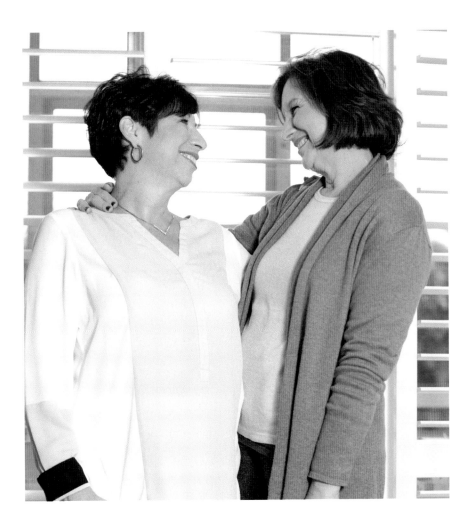

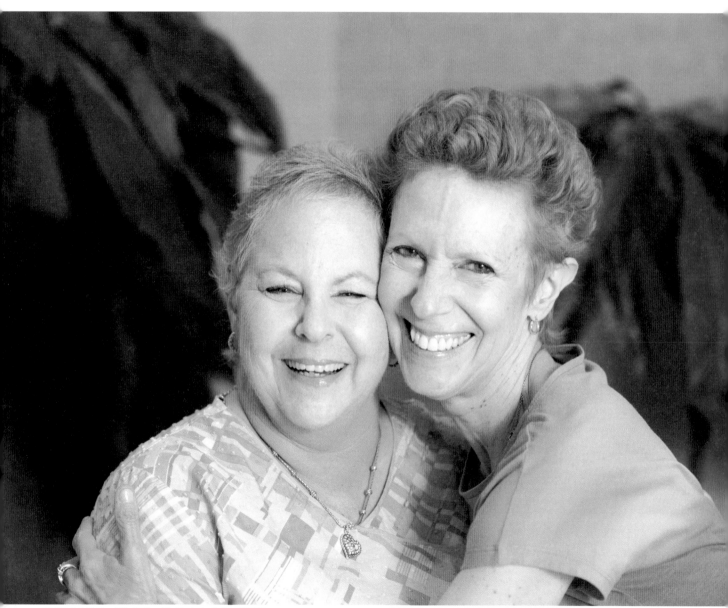

Kathy Ammirata, RN, OCN, with Marjorie Gelber [right]

The Unsung Hero

KATHY AMMIRATA, RN, OCN [FLORIDA CANCER CARE IN SUNRISE, FLORIDA]

WRITTEN BY MARJORIE GELBER

I AM NOT A WRITER or even a persuasive person, but I have gotten paid most of my professional career as an observer and listener; first as a school counselor, and, most recently, for more than 11 years, as a small group facilitator at Gilda's Club South Florida. More importantly for the task at hand, I am also a 13-year breast cancer survivor who has had the honor of observing and being cared for by the unsung hero and angel on earth, Kathy Ammirata.

IN MY CAPACITY as a facilitator in a cancer support community, I have heard countless stories about the skills of many wonderful oncology nurses as the members of Gilda's Club deal with all different kinds of cancer at an extensive number of hospitals and doctors' offices. I am amazed at the amount of compassion shown by these dedicated individuals. Yet, it always makes me appreciate how lucky I am to have Kathy for my own care.

I first met her in 2000 when I was initially diagnosed, and I was truly fortunate that she was working for my oncologist, Dr. Elizabeth Tan-Chiu, when I had my first recurrence in 2008. I have been receiving Herceptin infusions every three weeks since then, and am now on my third round of chemotherapy under Kathy's most compassionate and attentive eyes.

Why do I feel so strongly that Kathy is extraordinary? Not only is she the model of efficiency, hard work and tireless energy, but I have watched her over the years working kindly and patiently with all types of patients—from women in clinical trials who are worried about being "guinea pigs" to others who are angry at the world about their diagnosis, as well as those who are seriously depressed and have given up hope. Kathy approaches each of them as if they are her only patients. She'll look them in the eyes, hold their hands and talk compassionately with sincere "you-can-do-this" encouragement, even as they vent their frustrations.

It never ceases to impress upon me how even the most agitated patient will calm down after only a few minutes with Kathy, as she always seems to find just the right words with each of them. Yet, she is so humble! Even when being showered with gratitude, I have seen her smile, shrug her shoulders and say, "I'm just doing my job." And what a job she does. In all of the 13 years I've known her, I don't think I've ever seen her take a lunch break. I've joked with her that I think she's like the Energizer Bunny in sneakers and probably couldn't be more efficient if she wore roller skates instead!

I have seen her on numerous occasions work long after 5 p.m., making sure everyone is comfortable and well taken care of, even running after a patient who had left something behind. What amazes me even more is that after giving 110 percent during her full-time oncology nursing job with Dr. Tan-Chiu, she goes home every night to care for her wheelchair-bound adult son, then comes back to work each day with renewed sense of purpose and dedication.

I am also impressed that Kathy has such an excellent memory. She always takes the time to ask her patients about family members, and not just "How's your daughter?" but "How is Melanie doing in college?"

She is knowledgeable and up-to-date about an extensive amount of resources available for each patient. For example, she informs her patients about all the free programs offered by the American Cancer Society for wigs, make-up consultations and rides to treatment, and even keeps hats, scarves and wigs, as well as books, videos, reading materials and other donated items available in the chemo room for the convenience of her patients.

I have observed her numerous times as she talks with kindness and the utmost patience, especially as she gently explains (for probably the millionth time over the course of her career) what each "newbie" to chemotherapy might expect, sprinkling in suggested do's and don'ts, as well as helpful hints that the printed drug company literature might not include, in a way that somehow causes the "deer in the headlights" look to disappear from a woman's face.

She'll look them in the eyes, hold their hands and talk compassionately with sincere "you-can-do-this" encouragement, even as they vent their frustrations.

In fact, when I recently found out from Dr. Tan-Chiu that my breast cancer had recurred for the second time and I needed chemotherapy once again, I went right over to Kathy, who gave me a gentle, warm hug that was exactly what I needed. Sensing immediately that I did not want to dwell in "Pity City," Kathy instantly switched into her mode of "OK, this is what we need to do" and gave me her wonderful pep talk, as well as handing me the appropriate literature for me to take home and read about the chemotherapy drug I would be receiving.

My numerous questions came next and, as always, Kathy waited patiently as I wrote everything down. Before she went to take care of another patient, she trotted over to the nearby computer to reserve the appointments times that would best fit my schedule.

In her free time, Kathy participates in the Broward County Oncology Nursing Society and even asked me to attend one of their monthly meetings as someone who inspires others. I was very proud to stand up in front of all the other oncology nurses and brag about Kathy and not myself! After all the speeches were over, I was surprised how many other guests came over to me to share their admiration for Kathy, too.

It is my utmost pleasure to recommend Kathy Ammirata as the oncology nurse whose compassion, expertise and helpfulness has made all the difference in my cancer journey, as well as in the lives of many others! ❧

Above & Beyond

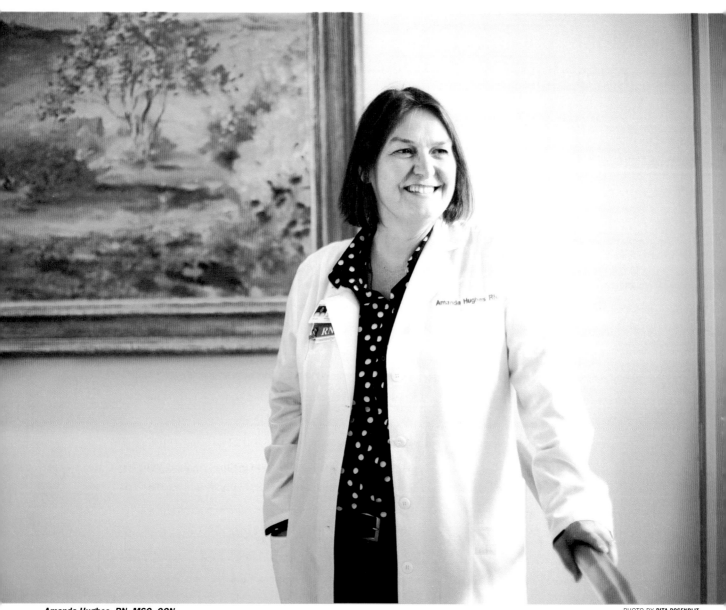

Amanda Hughes, RN, MSC, OCN

Cheerleader, Coach and Comedian

AMANDA HUGHES, RN, MSC, OCN

[MEMORIAL SLOAN KETTERING CANCER CENTER IN NEW YORK, NEW YORK]

WRITTEN BY KAYLEIGH R. COUPE

MANY TIMES IN LIFE, things take an unexpected turn. We plan our days and weeks and our whole lives in our minds. March 9, 2011, was one of those days for me; just a typical day in the life of Kayleigh Coupe.

Above & Beyond

BUT MARCH 9, 2011, ended up being the day my doctor told me I had cancer. Complicating things further, I was told I had a very rare tumor type and that local treatment was not going to be an option. After consulting with my family, we decided to go to Memorial Sloan Kettering Cancer Center.

When I had my first consult in New York, the doctor told me my prognosis was good since this rare tumor type was very treatable, with 85 percent responding well to the front-line chemotherapy regimen. But mine didn't. A few months after my chemotherapy had ended, the tumor recurred.

It was then I was referred to Dr. Darren Feldman at Sloan Kettering, and it was there I met Amanda Hughes, RN, MSC, OCN. I did not know it at that time, but Amanda would soon be much more to me than just another medical professional. Over the next four months, Amanda would at times become an extra parent, a cheerleader, a coach, a mentor and a comedian. I would soon realize I needed all of these in my life.

The next line of chemotherapy was a difficult one; high-dose chemotherapy with autologous stem cell transplant. This required me to live more than 200 miles from home and stay in New York during the four-month treatment cycle. Before treatment could start, I had to go through a procedure to harvest the oocytes from my ovaries as the high-dose chemotherapy could potentially destroy them. After that, my own blood stem cells would need to be collected, which required a central venous catheter (CVC) to be inserted. Finally, once enough blood stem cells were collected, the high-dose chemotherapy could begin.

Amanda was the medical compass that guided me through all of these procedures. Early on, all of this was very overwhelming and confusing. Each specialist had his or her own area to cover, but Amanda seemed to be the one person who could put it all together for me and explain what needed to be done, when it needed to be done, why it needed to be done and what I should expect. She was the one person who made me feel that I was still in control and yes, I can do this.

On many occasions, Amanda went the extra mile for me. One small example that was hugely important to me was her willingness to stop what she was doing to do a blood draw for me. My veins are very, very small, and it is always a major problem when a phlebotomist tries to do a blood draw. It takes longer than usual and after being poked with a needle many times, it is very painful. Blood could be easily drawn from the CVC, but a phlebotomist cannot do that, it requires an RN. Amanda volunteered that any time I needed blood drawn, I could ask them to call whatever floor she was on and she would come down and do the blood draw through my CVC. It seems small, but it was huge to me and she knew that.

Amanda also taught me to be as independent as possible, showing me how to properly do a sterile dressing change on my catheter and how to properly measure my outputs in the hospital so I did not need to have

TEACHING MOMENT:

Each specialist had his or her own area to cover, but Amanda seemed to be the one person who could put it all together for me and explain what needed to be done, when it needed to be done, why it needed to be done and what I should expect.

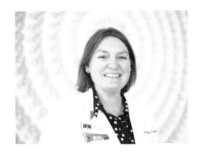

to call for assistance every time I wanted to use the bathroom. With the amount of hydration chemotherapy patients receive, visits to the bathroom are frequent. Again, these things may seem small, but when your entire world seems to be in the hands of others, every little piece of independence feels like a milestone towards winning the battle.

A few days after finishing a chemotherapy cycle, my platelet counts would be very low and I was susceptible to infection and would have difficulty clotting if any bleeding started. One day, as I was on my way to the clinic for hydration, I developed a nose bleed. I could not get the bleeding to stop, and I was soon convincing myself that this was serious, and I was probably going to die this way. When I finally arrived at the clinic in somewhat of a panic with several blood-soaked tissues around my nose, the first person to see me was Amanda. She simply looked at me and smiled and said, "Didn't your mother tell you not to pick your nose?" In an instant, I realized I was going to be all right after all.

My experience with Amanda over those four months in early 2012 gave me enough examples to fill 20 pages. She always reminded me of where I was in my treatment plan, how far I had come already and gave me strength and encouragement to continue all the way to win my battle with cancer. She was always reassuring, she was always smiling, she always got me the answer to my questions, she always had time for me and she was always there for me when I needed her. She never let me down. Sloan Kettering has over 12,000 employees, and for someone my age, such a huge organization can be overwhelming. Amanda made it easy and made it personal.

Cancer treatment interrupted my studies at nursing school. Now with my life back on track, I expect to become a registered nurse myself in the summer of 2014. Amanda's inspiration to me as a patient will soon serve as an inspiration in my goal to become a great nurse. In times of doubt, I only need to ask myself, "What would Amanda do?" ❧

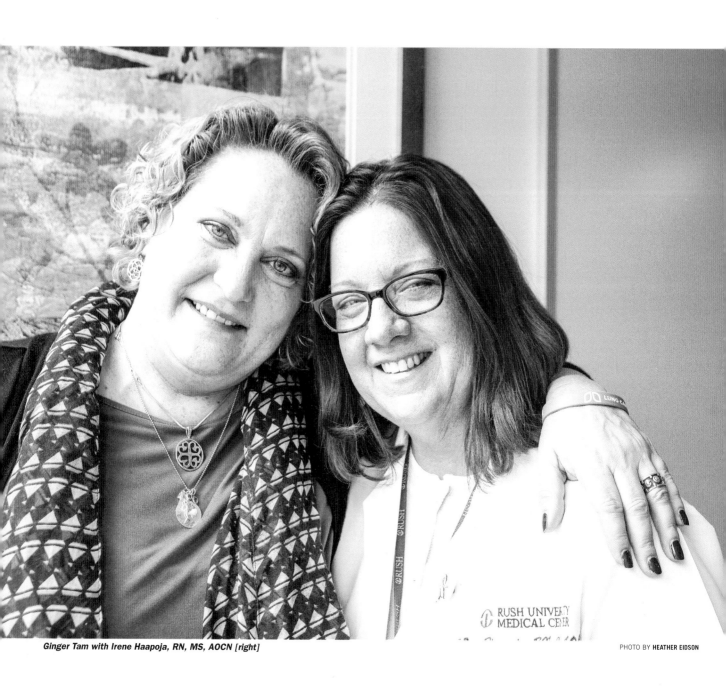

Ginger Tam with Irene Haapoja, RN, MS, AOCN [right]

Never Alone

IRENE HAAPOJA, RN, MS, AOCN [RUSH UNIVERSITY MEDICAL CENTER IN CHICAGO, ILLINOIS]

WRITTEN BY GINGER TAM

"ARE YOU HERE ALONE? Do you have any family with you?" the resident asked me. My heart began to beat faster. Yes, I was alone. I was always alone. I was the single mother of 7-year-old girl.

THE RESIDENT WENT ON TO SAY, "Your lung scan shows what seems to be metastatic disease." I didn't understand at first. "You mean you found a spot?" I asked. "Are you saying it's cancer? Could there be a mistake? Could it be pneumonia? A fungus?" I kept firing questions.

She looked at me and said, "I don't think so. There is just too much of it."

What did this mean? Was I going to die this week or next month? My worst nightmare had come true. That moment will be forever frozen in time. I can remember every single detail.

After that all I could say was, "Oh God, my daughter!"

I kept repeating it over and over, "Are you sure? My Lord, my daughter."

The resident sat there for a short while and then told me to wait while she paged the social worker. She then left me alone for what seemed an eternity. She had gone on to take care of other patients. I sat there in shock and alone with my heart breaking for my daughter and the pain she would have to endure. I was also the caregiver to my 84-year-old mother.

I began to panic and cry out, "God, please help me. What do I do now?"

Then, in a very small moment of clarity, I realized I was still sitting alone in room having just been told my lungs were full of cancer. At that moment I knew something was really wrong. Shouldn't someone be here with me telling me what we do now? That there is hope?

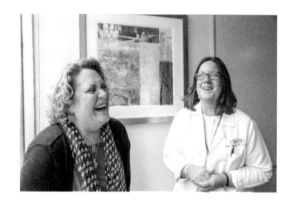

I realized I needed to get out of there. I knew I wanted to fight, and I had to find the right place to do it. I had to fight for my daughter. I walked out alone in slow motion, and I never looked back.

That same night, I called a friend to sit with me. She told me about a doctor at Rush University Medical Center, Dr. Philip Bonomi, one of the top oncologists in the country. I made an appointment for the next day.

From the moment I set foot at Rush, I was never alone again. I met Irene who saw and understood my unique circumstances. She made sure I knew their team was going to fight this with me. She gave me her cell phone number and said call anytime.

She also had a daughter about the same age as mine. She showed sincere concern for her, as well as me. She made sure I had friends to help me at home and my mother while she set me up with counseling right away. The counselor was in the room within five minutes.

Irene Haapoja, RN, AOCN, I prefer to call her advanced practitioner, sets the bar with her knowledge and expertise. With a cancer diagnosis, we all know the timing in which we receive treatment can be critical. Whenever my treatment was threatened by insurance, the problem would somehow miraculously disappear.

TEACHING MOMENT:

Irene sees a big part of her job as keeping her patients from having any stress.

I knew Irene had gotten on the phone and worked her magic. She never gave me a minute to worry about it.

I remember one day going for chemo and was told my insurance was canceled. Irene didn't flinch. I don't know how she did it but she made sure I did not leave that day without treatment.

When I needed clinical trials, Irene gave me insight and made sure they happened. Her knowledge of how the system works was invaluable. Irene made sure all of my records and the proper paperwork were done correctly and on time even if it meant working on her days off.

When the screening process on a trial did not go well, I was sent home to let my cancer progress more. I lost the last open slot in the country that day. The next slot would not be available for months, and that was too long for me.

Irene suggested I contact all the sites with that trial and try to get on a waiting list. The next day I tried the sites directly, and found one that was adding a spot that day! They had just gotten an email from the sponsoring drug company as I was calling. If it hadn't been for Irene, I would have missed that.

As a single mom, having enough on my plate, any of these things could have caused me enormous stress. But Irene sees a big part of her job as keeping her patients from having any stress. I have never seen her anything but calm. Even in crisis she doesn't change. I think she just moves a little faster. I am convinced it is a special gene, of which I certainly do not have, or she is an angel.

She made it possible for my daughter to set up a table at a fundraising event to sell Rainbow Loom bracelets for lung cancer awareness. She knew how important it was to have Amelia, my daughter, involved in my healing process.

Irene held my hand through it all and still does. There have been hundreds of phone calls and texts over the past three years. On my tough days, she lets me cry and reassures me there will be another plan when we need it. On my good days, we laugh together. If I don't call or text for a couple of weeks, which almost never happens, she will send me a text and ask me, "Don't you love me anymore?"

Being a single mom facing the fight for my life against stage 4 lung cancer, I don't know how I would have done this without Irene. I wish we all could have advocates and friends like her. Thanks to her, I am never alone. ❧

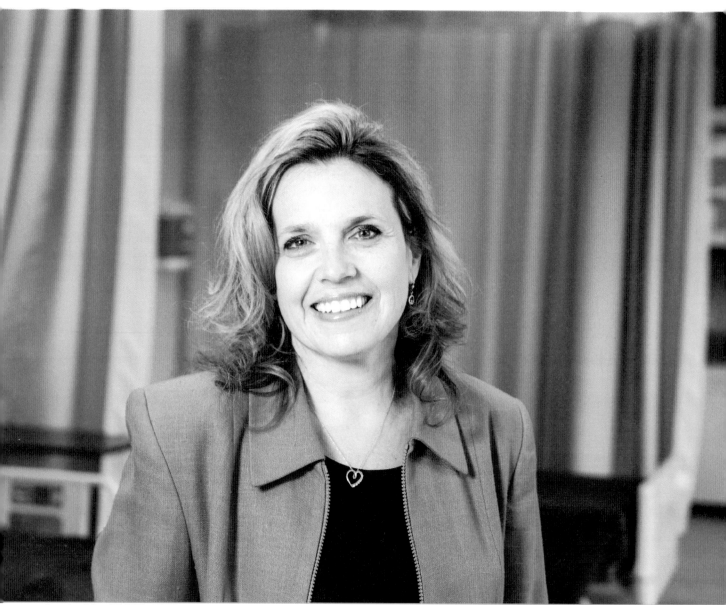

Jeannine Arias, RN, MSN, AOCNS

Beyond an Extraordinary Healer

JEANNINE ARIAS, RN, MSN, AOCNS [ADVENTIST MIDWEST HEALTH IN HINSDALE, ILLINOIS]

WRITTEN BY DIANE T. HUSTON

I FIRST MET JEANNINE ARIAS, RN, in 1985 when we started working in the ICU at Morris Hospital, a small community hospital in Morris, Illinois. She was fresh out of her nursing program and much like a sponge, wanting to soak in every piece of knowledge afforded to her at the small hospital. However, I knew she was destined for something far greater than what this small hospital could offer her, and two years later, we both left for Chicago where she flourished in the nursing arena. Ultimately, our career paths diverged in 1990 when I was commissioned in the Air Force, but we still kept in touch through the years.

JEANNINE FURTHERED her education as a master's-prepared professional nurse and flourished with over 28 years of hospital experience, including leadership roles in administration, oncology, emergency and critical care nursing. As a visionary leader with a passion for advancement of the nursing profession and a talent for empowering collaborative efforts in program growth, while being responsive to customer satisfaction coupled with alignment to drive the best practices and patient outcomes, she has been the associate clinical director of oncology and navigational services since April 2012 at Adventist Midwest Health in Illinois. Since being a vital entity of this four-hospital region, Jeannine has written and secured grants of $332,000 for prehabilitation to provide services at the time of diagnosis for high-risk cancer patients; $25,000 for colon cancer screening and prevention in DuPage County; and an ongoing Open Arms Fund for breast

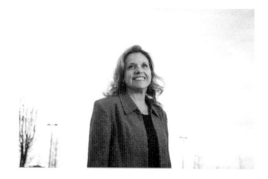

cancer screening and prevention. Furthermore, she has published three articles on breast cancer in the *Journal of Oncology Navigation and Survivorship*. This woman is phenomenal with her benevolence to promote the best health care access to uninsured and underinsured patients in DuPage County, while ensuring the patients have up-to-date information and securing additional resources as the situation dictates.

She never stops visualizing how to improve the outcomes of cancer patients. Jeannine is at the forefront of the new Adventist Cancer Institute, a state-of-the-art 54,000 square foot cancer center showcasing the regional interdisciplinary oncology services to better meet the patients' needs. She was key to the development of the navigation program from the ground up, introduced six new programs and contributed to the increase, in two years, from 9 percent nurse certification to 87 percent for nursing magnet and breast/oncology accreditation.

Through these endeavors, she has positively promoted the physicians' perception for the need of a navi-

TEACHING MOMENT:

She was key to the development of the navigation program from the ground up...

gation program on behalf of their patients. In addition to these accomplishments, Jeannine presented Adventist Cancer Institute's navigational outcomes to the Academy of Oncology Nurse and Patient Navigators conference the past two years. Finally, she was invited as a member of the National Consortium of Breast Centers task force to assist in the development of national navigation exams and build the national navigation conference center agendas.

I could write volumes of what this woman has forged in the field of being an extraordinary healer, but that is not the reason I am submitting her nomination. I am a grateful one-year survivor of stage 4A oropharyngeal cancer. Having gone through the ordeal of first hearing the words "positive for squamous cell cancer" to "no metabolic activity noted" on the PET scan after 35 doses of IMRT, 3 rounds of cisplatin and a few setbacks along the way, that year after being diagnosed was a total blur.

I had excellent health care providers where I received treatment from the receptionist to the social worker and all the other partners along the way. My caregivers were with me every minute during this most difficult period. Because of them, I am here today to submit this. However, my treatment center does not have a navigational program in place. I knew what I was to accomplish during the treatment phase, but post-treatment, I was unaware of what would happen next.

Through *CURE*, I learned the concept of a navigation program and follow-up, developing my own through researching my disease process and finding a support group. I wish I had been a part of Jeannine's program; I might not have felt so alone.

It is the navigation program that is crucial for the survivors and their caregivers and families to get back to some type of normalcy after hearing those dreadful words of being diagnosed with cancer. I know that, without a doubt, Jeannine's integral day-to-day involvement at the new Adventist Cancer Institute will do just that for the patients and their families in DuPage County. She is an amazing leader, yet still keeps her finger on the pulse of caring. Jeannine is that extraordinary healer! ❧

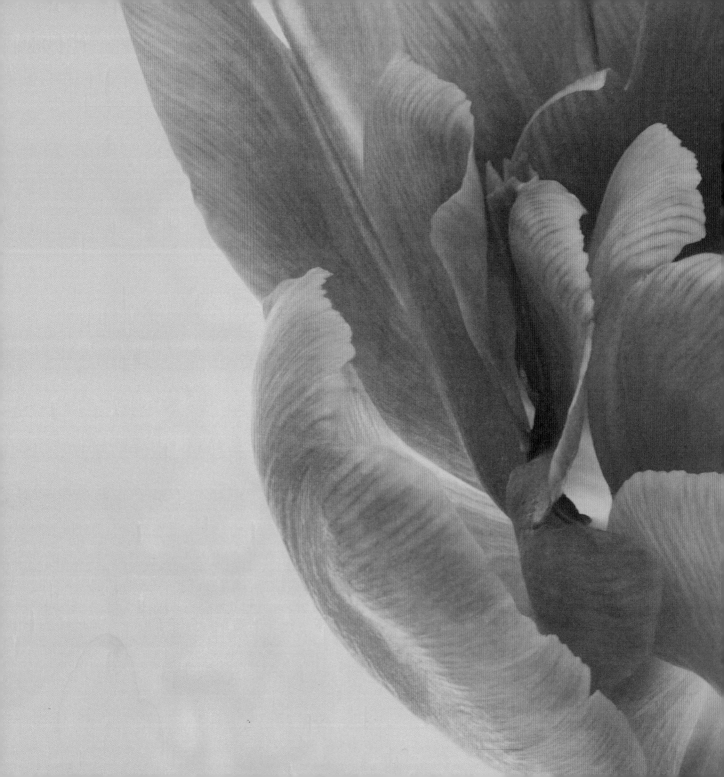

CHAPTER 2

Peer Tribute

My Extraordinary Healer

KATINA WILSON, RN, BSN, OCN [FLORIDA HOSPITAL CELEBRATION IN CELEBRATION, FLORIDA]

WRITTEN BY HOLLY JOHNSON, MD

WHEN I THINK OF HEALING, I think of good health and well-being even in the presence of disease. Healing is the recovery of the heart and soul. We are all healers of the world no matter who we are. We are here because we can make a difference.

WHEN WE LIVE from the heart and therefore bless another person, this moment of blessing becomes a moment of expansion and helps us to discover ourselves. When someone sees our potential, we have an experience of self-worth. When we experience self-worth, we can find meaning and purpose, and through meaning, we can transform our life experiences, even with cancer. In *Kitchen Table Wisdom*, Dr. Rachel Naomi Remen writes, "When we are blessed, we are led through a one-way door and there is no looking back."

When I think of extraordinary people in my life with the power to heal and to bless, I think of Nurse Katina Wilson. I met Katina when I, the doctor, became a cancer patient. Five years ago, after finding a mass on my own chest X-ray, my chest was cracked open and I was diagnosed with Hodgkin's lymphoma.

On my first day of chemotherapy, I sat in a brown La-Z-Boy chair in a common room with other patients ready to be hooked up to their cancer-fighting cocktails. I was strong and confident, yet bewildered and scared at the same time. Katina was handpicked to be my nurse. She walked over to me, smiled at me, put my small, cool hand in her big, warm hand and simply said, "I'm Katina. I am going to be your nurse. Leave everything to me."

As she reached over to access my port for the first time and my first drip was ready to roll, I lost all control as reality slapped me in the face–I have cancer! I am about to receive chemo. This can't be happening! Katina took this emotional outburst in stride, hugged me, held me and reassured me that I was OK. This was the moment she first healed me.

There are so many ways we heal others. We can heal each other through the simple words we say, the smile we share, the eye contact we make and the prayers we pray. Katina is naturally quietly awesome at these simple things. She is a healer through her service and heart for her patients. She is gentle with her touch, skilled in the way she gives care and would do anything to make a cancer patient's experience a better one.

When one of my chemo posse couldn't afford her medications, Katina applied for and was granted money for this patient to receive the care she needed.

When my chemo posse made her a birthday cake, she was the one who sliced it up and passed out the plates. When I brought a family member or friend with me for support, she made sure they had a chair and a hug too. She performed wonders with her words to comfort my husband and family and friends who accompanied me to my treatments.

Katina heals not only through her heart, but also through her feet, on her own time. In 2010, she raised $2,800 for Susan G. Komen and walked the Susan G. Komen 3-Day 60-mile trek to benefit breast cancer research and awareness.

Nurse Wilson is striving to become a better healer through her continuing education. Katina is so committed to being her best–to give her best to others–that she became a nursing stu-

TEACHING MOMENT:

She is gentle with her touch, skilled in the way she gives care and would do anything to make a cancer patient's experience a better one.

dent for the second time in her life and is now enrolled in the Dual Oncology & Adult-Gerontology Nurse Practitioner program at the University of South Florida. Due to her commitment to excellence and patient care in 2013, she was awarded the American Cancer Society's graduate nursing scholarship. She expects to graduate in spring 2016. Her ultimate goal is to obtain her doctorate in nursing, which I have no doubt she will accomplish with a huge smile on her face and a few of her biggest fans—her survivors—in the audience.

Katina saw the potential and life force in my special chemo posse and called all of us her VIPs. She understands that to help and care for humans in the tender way we need to be, she must first be human. As our bodies betrayed us, she helped each of us to try to find meaning and purpose in our diagnosis. She met each of us exactly where we were at with our own limitations and understanding of what was happening to us.

One of my last memories I have of Katina being my nurse was at my last infusion. I walked into the chemo room bedecked in my cowgirl hat, comfy khaki pants and loose shirt so she could easily access my port. As I came around the corner to my chair, I heard sounds of Gloria Gaynor's "I Will Survive."

Katina and the other nurses lined up, grabbed my arm and we all started line dancing in celebration of the big finish and being cancer free! Other patients clapped along, and again Katina healed me. Thanks to my extraordinary healer, I walked through a blessed survivor's one-way door, and since then, there has been no looking back. ❧

Why She Matters So Much

TERESA GONZALEZ, RN [KAISER PERMANENTE, SOUTH BAY MEDICAL CENTER, IN HARBOR CITY, CALIFORNIA]

WRITTEN BY PAULA VINCENT, RN, CNM

IT'S HARD TO FIND a silver lining when you've been told you have cancer for the second time. This is my life now. I hold tight to the belief that I am a survivor who is living with, not dying from, metastatic breast cancer. This helps provide the balance, hope and gratitude I try to find in every moment and with each person who is a part of my life and recovery.

MOST ARE FAMILIAR AND CONSTANT, others newer and less certain. After being diagnosed in April of 2012, I decided to pursue aggressive treatment at my local hospital. My initial impressions of the oncology unit and staff left me feeling uncertain and anxious, as I found myself comparing the stellar care I had received on the East Coast with my first breast cancer diagnosis 14 years earlier. I felt let down. As a practicing clinician for close to 30 years, I have to admit that I have very high standards for the care I give, as well as receive.

Within a short time after starting treatment, I realized the "fit" wasn't right with both the oncologist I had been assigned to and the oncology nurse that had been caring for me. I knew this time around that I needed to be both mentally and physically prepared for the hardest battle I had ever fought, and l knew with even more certainty I needed a team of warriors who would always be by my side throughout treatments that would never finish.

Enter Teresa.

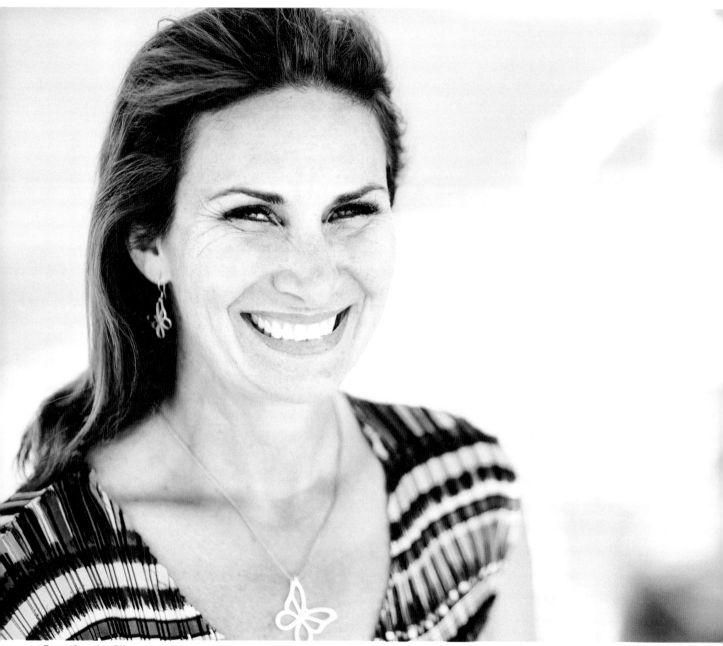

Teresa Gonzalez, RN

Within the first few minutes of meeting her, I knew on a deep level that she was a perfect fit, a kindred spirit. This continues to be the case after nearly two years. There are so many qualities that come together to make Teresa unique and special.

From the beginning, her professionalism and expertise in oncology care was evident, and this put me at ease as I came to understand and accept my need to let go of control and trust her to do the job she knew so well how to do. Her personality was much like my own: strong-willed, intelligent, focused, competent and efficient, with a big dose of kindness and compassion to soften the edges.

I felt, and still feel, safe in her care, and this allows me to return again and again for the treatment I dread but so desperately need. Each Monday and Tuesday when I arrive for my blood work and chemotherapy, I am greeted with her warm and welcoming smile, and her never-ending array of eclectic, brightly colored scrub uniforms, quirky socks and festive caps.

I learned early on that she has great adoration for the Winnie-the-Pooh character Tigger, whose plush animals, stickers and other accoutrements don her personal nurse's supply cart. I feel my spirits lift when I hear her rolling cart make its way down the hallway toward my room, with bouncy and smiling Teresa following closely behind. She almost always saves me one of the coveted large treatment rooms, where I settle in as she welcomes my support people, dims the overhead lights, and offers me water and hot tea, a warm blanket and words of encouragement.

Her intuition allows for the right balance of a comforting presence, without being overly intrusive. She knows the details of my care and treatment, but never fails to check and recheck my information and treatment protocol to ensure safety and accuracy. With each visit, she reviews my day-to-day symptoms and remedies, lab values, treatment plans and upcoming appointments. Teresa has been known to call and check in on me at home with new lab results, after an especially hard chemo day or when I've received difficult news.

Our relationship has seasoned, and over time, Teresa and I have begun opening up to one another. Me sharing my fears, sadness and uncertainties with being a mother of three with advanced cancer, and she with the loss and grief she lives with after losing her brother to cancer last year. I deeply believe these experiences, although hard to give voice to, have allowed us to transcend a level of intimacy and caring that flows directly into the work she does with me, as well as many other patients who are equally fortunate to be cared for by this incredible woman.

When Teresa has a day off, or happens to be assigned to another patient on the same day I have my treatment, things just don't feel the same for me. This is not to say that the other nursing staff are not competent or qualified, there is simply no one who comes close to replacing her. I have the utmost respect and gratitude for her presence in my life and for the many gifts she shares by just being her wonderful self. For this, I remain grateful and feel blessed that we are sharing this cancer journey together. She deserves every recognition for her excellent and compassionate oncology nursing care, and for being one of my lifelines.

These things, and more, are why she matters so much. ✖

TEACHING MOMENT:

From the beginning, her professionalism and expertise in oncology care was evident, and this put me at ease as I came to understand and accept my need to let go of control and trust her to do the job she knew so well how to do.

Healing Over Decades

JOANNE CANDELA, RN, ANP-BC

[MEMORIAL SLOAN KETTERING CANCER CENTER IN NEW YORK, NEW YORK]

WRITTEN BY STACIE CORCORAN, MS, RN, AOCNS

OVER MY 25 YEARS as an oncology nurse, I have had the privilege of working with many talented and dedicated clinicians. However, certain individuals stand out as being truly special because they bring a completely different level of professionalism and humanity to their interactions with peers and care of patients. Joanne Candela is such a person. Her unmatched compassion, integrity and commitment to her patients make her a truly deserving recipient of the *CURE* Extraordinary Healer Award.

I FIRST HAD the pleasure of meeting Joanne three years ago when I became her supervisor as nurse leader for the Survivorship Program at Memorial Sloan Kettering Cancer Center. Working as a survivorship nurse practitioner (NP) at Sloan Kettering, Joanne cares for a very complicated group of patients—young adult survivors and the adult survivors of pediatric cancers. The complex set of long-term and late effects experienced by these patients (which vary in terms of onset and severity) impact not only physical health, but also psychological well-being and social development. Monitoring for and managing the complicated late effects of chemotherapy, radiotherapy and surgery require astute assessment, detailed follow-up care and sophisticated coordination of services.

Joanne's in-depth understanding of post-treatment effects such as cardiac disease, endocrine dysfunction and risk for second malignancies is essential to the timely identification and management of these serious and sometimes life-threatening issues.

But Joanne does not limit her practice to the medical management of these complex patients; rather, she works with each to address such critically important issues as employment, insurance coverage and social integration with peers. She is an expert at guiding them to local and national available resources. Joanne's focus is on healing, an especially important and unique process for childhood cancer survivors that requires attention to immediate problems, anticipation of potential future issues, interventions and education to promote optimal physical and psychological function.

Joanne's focus is on healing, an especially important and unique process for childhood cancer survivors that requires attention to immediate problems, anticipation of potential future issues, interventions and education to promote optimal physical and psychological function.

On par with Joanne's exceptional clinical skills is her ability to establish trust and confidence with her patients. Their unending praise and appreciation for her skill and commitment provide some insight into the difference she has made in so many lives. Patients have commented, "Thank you, thank you. You have no idea the difference that you make in my life;" "As always, thanks for your attention and follow-up advice. You make it easy, and that is no small gift;" and "I could not do this without you!"

Her attending physician colleagues write, "Needless to say, the patients love her. Joanne is a NP without parallel. I would not hesitate to entrust my dearest family members to her care;" "Joanne is remarkably dedicated to her patients and has a commitment to health and welfare that supersedes her everyday clinical responsibilities. She's worked to address recent changes in Medicaid coverage, which have helped improve access to much needed care for poor or uninsured cancer survivors."

Medical residents have acknowledged the insight gained through clinical rotations with Joanne, stating,

"We spend much of our time in the hospital, working with sick, active treatment patients. I got to see the other side of cancer care, and what patients experience in the long-term, follow-up setting.

Observing how Joanne practices has given me perspective on what I'm working toward with my own patients. This rich experience has made me more comfortable with them. Joanne's devotion to her patients is evident, and she serves as a role model for young clinicians striving to be caring and understanding providers through excellent clinical care and bedside manner."

Nursing colleagues praise the calm demeanor and empathy Joanne brings to each patient. They comment on her resourcefulness and ability to solve problems, stating, "Joanne is a wonderful, motivational mentor. She is always imparting new knowledge she's gained through reading or attending conferences to her nursing colleagues and other members of the healthcare team. She always has the answer to an obscure question! She inspires our entire team to learn, question current practices and grow."

At our holiday gathering this past year, Joanne told a story of a patient she cared for on the pediatric inpatient unit at MSK in her first month working as a new nurse. Her young patient was a 14-day-old newborn diagnosed with a neuroblastoma. Joanne described her initial feelings of fear and doubt, which eventually gave way to hope. She included the new mother as much as possible in the baby's care, and formed a bond with this mother that would prove fateful many years later. With tears in her eyes, Joanne described the phone call she had received earlier that day from this former patient, now a woman in her 30s, grappling with endocrine and cardiac dysfunction. After all these years, the bond that had been formed between the new, terrified mother and the new (also terrified) nurse served to reunite this patient with her oncology nurse. Through her mother's guidance, the patient reached out to Joanne to care for her once again. Not surprisingly, Joanne assisted the patient in navigating insurance issues and was ultimately able to see her in clinic and begin addressing her medical problems, again becoming the nurse caring for the patient she had first known as a newborn.

Intelligent, thoughtful and generous are qualities that come up repeatedly in talking with Joanne's patients and colleagues. As a committed educator, collaborator and caregiver, Joanne has influenced and improved the lives of many, many cancer survivors. A role model for all oncology providers, both inexperienced and seasoned, Joanne reminds us why we chose this field and of how privileged we are to care for our patients and contribute to their healing every step of the way. ❧

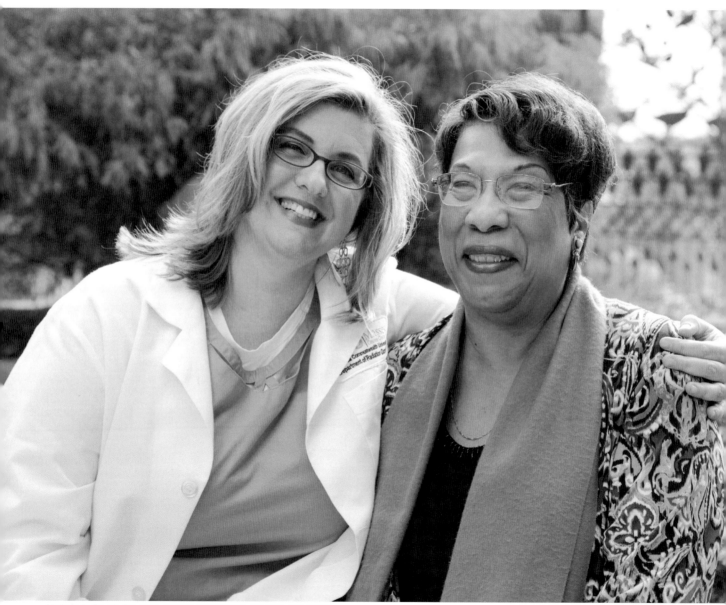

Melinda B. Roach, RN, BSN, with Diane Crawford, RN, BSN, CIC [right]

A True Patient Advocate and Holistic Caregiver

MELINDA B. ROACH, RN, BSN

[VIRGINIA COMMONWEALTH UNIVERSITY MASSEY CANCER CENTER IN RICHMOND, VIRGINIA]

WRITTEN BY DIANE CRAWFORD, RN, BSN, CIC

I BELIEVE that cancer has a way of showing up just when other troubles are present or brewing.

FOR INSTANCE, AFTER 20 YEARS as an infection control nurse with advance training and certification, I was forced into what I term, "economic retirement." Next, on Dec. 6, 2012, I lost my beloved 14-year-old pet, a Maltese canine, to Cushing's disease. Maybe both losses were inevitable, but they were no less disheartening to me.

Finally, by the end of that December, I received notification that my annual mammogram was somewhat abnormal and requiring follow up. I thought, "This can't be anything serious; it's only been a year since my last normal screening." How devastating it was to get that confirmed breast biopsy report of a malignant tumor in my left breast in March 2013.

I felt like my world was caving in on me. I've been a registered nurse for 34 years and, for the first time, I found myself in a panic. At times I was confused or indecisive concerning my health and future. Would anyone be there to understand and help me in my struggles? Who would help me manage the many silent feelings regarding breast cancer? More frightening, would I passively be treated like the nurse who should know it all?

In May, I did well through surgery, even though I ended up having a partial mastectomy instead of the lumpectomy. No chemotherapy was needed at this time, but radiation would be next. I was fortunate to qualify for brachytherapy radiation. However, it still was an unfamiliar procedure, and I was very anxious about short- and long-term side effects and discomforts. I didn't have a clue as to how well I would tolerate the procedure.

In early June, as I was registering in the VCU Massey Cancer Center's radiation oncology clinic, I met Mrs. Melinda (Mel) B. Roach, RN, prior to my being prepared for radiation treatment. Mel was very pleasant with a caring, relaxed and confident approach. She demonstrated familiarity with infection control techniques. If there's one thing that makes an infection control nurse relax and remain calm, it's to see caregivers utilizing the standard principles while rendering care. During the minor procedure of installing a balloon catheter in my breast by the physicians, she was attentive and explained the procedures to me. The administration of the radiation was to start in two days. I thought, "I hope things continue to go this well." Looks like positive first impressions certainly matter when it comes to reassuring patients.

On Monday morning, Mel greeted me with an enthusiastic attitude. Her approach made me feel safe and allowed me to concentrate on myself and getting better. It had been awhile since I only considered my well-being. She asked me if I needed something to help me relax while I lay isolated in the room during my radiation treatment. I said, "Since there is a CD player in here, what kind of music is available?" I really didn't think I could or would be accommodated. By the first radiation session, I got to listen to smooth jazz. The treatment was painless and time seemed to breeze by, but something was missing.

The second day of my radiation treatment, I felt a certain comfort level and trust in Mel. I asked Mel if there were any gospel CDs available. That afternoon, even with her hectic schedule,

TEACHING MOMENT:

I was cared for as a whole human being, as a patient as well as a nurse, who could express moments of sadness and anxiety and resolve them. I felt blessed to experience such genuine, protected and holistic care.

she got two gospel CDs from somewhere. As I listened to uplifting spiritual music, I started recognizing my blessings. I felt my burdens and past pains diminishing. At this point, nothing was more important than my fight against this cancer. I relaxed so deeply that a few times the radiation team monitoring me from the window (outer parameters of the radiation field) called my name to make sure I was all right or "still alive."

I thank God for placing Mrs. Roach into His plan of care. She certainly supported my spiritual needs at every session. No detail was too small for her attention. She arranged the twice-daily, five-day treatment schedule with consideration of my transportation issues and other medical needs.

When I expressed a desire to speak to a social worker, all I had to do was ask Mel. I was cared for as a whole human being, as a patient as well as a nurse, who could express moments of sadness and anxiety and resolve them. I felt blessed to experience such genuine, protected and holistic care.

In my entire years of nursing experience, I realized that it was a rarity to run into a nurse with such defined traits of a true patient advocate and holistic caregiver. I will never take such total quality care for granted. ❧

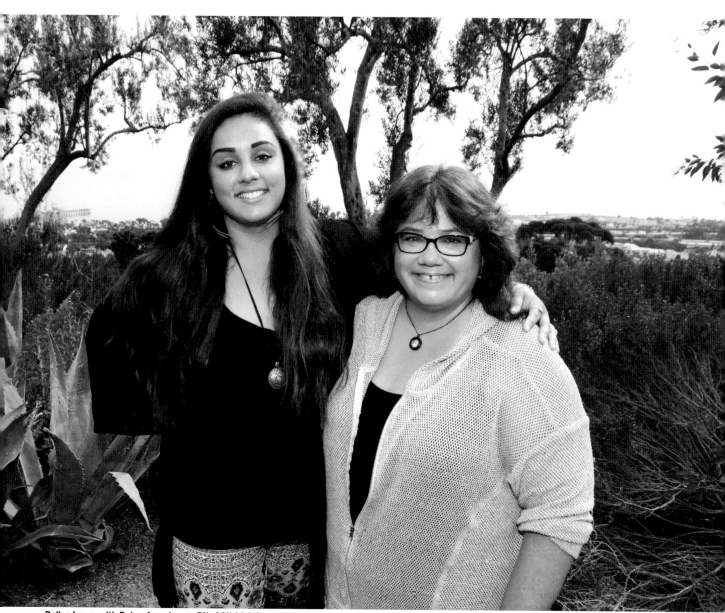

Dallas Lawry with Debra Anne Lawry, RN, OCN [right]

The Humblest Hero

DEBRA ANNE LAWRY, RN, OCN

WRITTEN BY DALLAS LAWRY

THERE IS A POEM by the author Linda Ellis called "The Dash," which refers to the dates on a tombstone, from the beginning to the end.

…

So, when your eulogy is being read,

with your life's actions to rehash…

would you be proud of the things they say

about how you spent YOUR dash?

…

A DASH. A tiny little line that, at the last sentence of your story, represents you entire life. Debra Lawry is the type of person that has taken her dash and touched too many lives to count.

Debbie is that nurse whom patients stop in the grocery store and say, "Do you remember me? You helped me through my chemo." She is that nurse whom peers say, "You always work at 200 percent, and I don't know how you do it." She is that nurse that walks with her survivors at Relay For Life, including her own mother, a breast cancer survivor. She is a patient advocate who has lobbied multiple times on Capitol Hill for the betterment of drug trials and affordability of chemotherapy. She is a bright smile and a loud burst of laughter. She is genuine, she is authentic, and she is an oncology nurse that has changed my life.

I am not a patient. I am not even a cancer survivor. But I have known Debbie for my entire life, and to say that she is a selfless caregiver with the heart of an oncology nurse, is the utmost understatement.

Since the day she earned her nursing degree, she has worked in the field of oncology, and has dedicated her entire life to it. Starting at St. John's Hospital in Oxnard, California, she spent about 20 years with the Ventura County Hematology Oncology Specialists, making her way from the acute oncology setting to the ambulatory care setting. She is currently working towards her master's degree in nursing education in order to train the next generation of nurses to be brilliant and compassionate patient advocates. She has also taken a firm leadership role in her field and is an esteemed oncology nurse educator for Amgen.

But she didn't always live in the world where cancer was no longer a death sentence. Debbie is from the time before growth factors and monoclonal antibodies. She has watched the promising practice of oncology become a world of hope and has just fallen even more in love with it.

Debbie doesn't use any of these words to describe herself. She is an exceptional leader and looked to as an expert nurse in the field, but she would never admit to it. She has earned numerous awards for her excellent patient care and work with Amgen, but would never tell anyone. She has planned entire Oncology Nursing Society symposiums for small chapters seeking help. But her greatest pride in the world is truly knowing that she has made a difference.

Debbie's humility is sometimes upsetting. I want her to know how phenomenal she is and how many people view her as a mentor, including myself. She has taught me that the most rewarding thing about oncology nursing is not all the plaques and the state-of-the-art research, it's the face of a patient who is truly at peace. It is the tears of a patient who has won the fight. It's the subtle smile in a patient's last breath. This is who Debbie truly is, the humblest of heroes.

She has shared the laughs and wiped the tears of cancer patients for the past 26 years. Most people only see the direct patient care side of oncology nursing, but Debbie has done all of it. The side that only few people see is the fearless leaders who set out to make a difference on a larger scale. She is a firm believer in clinical trials, in getting the best drugs to the patients when they need them most. She has stood on Capitol Hill fighting for these patients as they are at home battling their diseases. She knows the ethics of end-of-life care and educates on it. She has a strong desire to shape the future of nursing, and this is the driving force behind her going back to school. Debbie encompasses all aspects of the field of oncology, and in every single way, she strives for the best cancer care the United States can offer. She has truly dedicated her entire life to oncology.

"Cancer" is one of the most devastating words a patient and family can hear. It is truly an art to turn such a shocking and damaging diagnosis into an attitude of hope and strength. It is one thing to cure a disease, it's another thing to cure a person, but it's Debra Lawry who humbly does both.

It is always such a privilege to meet people who truly live each day of their life with the sole purpose of making a difference in the world. But it is an honor to call that person your mother.

On May 9, 2014, I was pinned into the nursing profession by my mom. I am so proud to follow in the footsteps of someone so humble yet so extraordinary, to be pinned into such a rewarding profession by someone who has truly been an exemplary oncology nurse. ❧

TEACHING MOMENT:

She has taught me that the most rewarding thing about oncology nursing is not all the plaques and the state-of-the-art research, it's the face of a patient who is truly at peace.

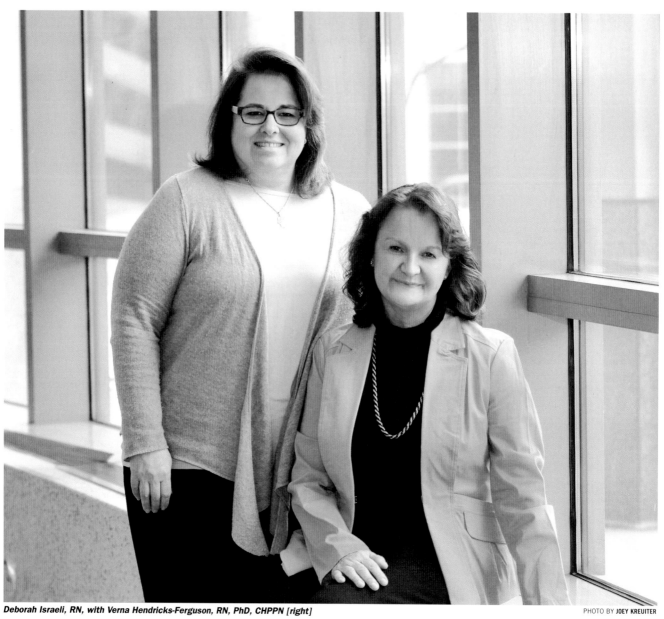

Deborah Israeli, RN, with Verna Hendricks-Ferguson, RN, PhD, CHPPN [right]

If Hurricanes Can Be Named, Why Can't Earthquakes Get One Too?

VERNA HENDRICKS-FERGUSON, RN, PHD, CHPPN

[SAINT LOUIS UNIVERSITY SCHOOL OF NURSING IN ST. LOUIS, MISSOURI]

WRITTEN BY DEBORAH ISRAELI, RN

DR. VERNA HENDRICKS-FERGUSON is an absolute inspiration to many others and me. When I started to think of all the ways she has impacted not only me, but also those in her care, all the work and studies and reports conducted and written, honestly, I don't think I could have fit it all in with the allowable word limit. I am thrilled to have the pleasure to share with you the weight that this slight woman has placed on me.

I HAVE BEEN A NURSE for more than 20 years and have had many mentors and influences in my life, but Dr. Hendricks-Ferguson's has been profound. When I decided to go back to school, my father had passed away a few years before that from pancreatic cancer. It piqued my interest in oncology. But, you know, I was a surgical nurse that was never going to change. When I walked into the class, I had no idea of who Dr. Hendricks-Ferguson was or the things she had done, especially in oncology.

She has a subtle energy. She does not need to be boisterous in her enthusiasm about what she does. It's enchanting, absolutely mesmerizing and draws you near to understand and appreciate her knowledge of oncology nursing and art of nursing care. It's so powerful. I learned that a whisper, a quiet voice, is very commanding. If you know me, that's just not my style. What a revelation!

In her nursing classes, we discussed the nurse's role, the percussion that nurses can have on their patients. I was magnetized by Dr. Hendricks-Ferguson's interest and passion for children with cancer in pain and the impact it had on their family and the world around them. Her work and her dedication have caused me to rethink my choice about going into oncology nursing. It went from a lukewarm interest to a girl-on-fire, full-throttle feeling about my desire to do this. She has shown me there is clarity in the quiet moments, power in a dignified death and peace with "walking" an oncology patient, their family and friends either toward wellness or death.

Dr. Hendricks-Ferguson is very comfortable speaking to nursing students about the needs of oncology patients, and she actively listens to what nursing students have to share. Hearing and listening are quite different. Listening is so much more intimate. When I was in class, she was always open to conversation, never rushing anyone through their process. That kind of patience is respect. One look at her CV and you can see how invested she is in her work, otherwise you would never know it. Dr. Hendricks-Ferguson is probably the most humble person I know. She has integrity; you can totally trust what she says. She is thorough and thoughtful. When she says that she will respond to an email or phone call, she does and her answers and opinions are well constructed. You will never get short shrift from Dr. Hendricks-Ferguson. She is attentive and genuinely warm. You always feel like you are her primary concern, the only person in the room.

Maybe it's hokey to sing such high praises about just one person. I can be an eye roller when someone talks about a "life-changing" event. I even mutter, "Oh, boy" under my breath. I've been told I have a pretty good "phony meter." I never, ever got this feeling from Dr. Hendricks-Ferguson. Her work is true and her compassion and passion for what she does is exemplary. I want to be her.

So, here's the upshot. Have you ever felt an earthquake, just a tremor? That is Dr. Hendricks-Ferguson; it is seemingly small in the earthquake realm. Not all earthquakes are destructive, quite the contrary. An earthquake can create and move mountains; change the course of major rivers (very stubborn rivers). I am happy and proud

TEACHING MOMENT:

Her work is true and her compassion and passion for what she does is exemplary.

to say that not only am I quite content in my choice to go into oncology nursing, but I have made strides in my nursing career. I have gone from being a floor nurse to working in a chemotherapy center and have recently accepted a position with Siteman Cancer Center as a nurse coordinator in the division of gynecology oncology. That kind of influence, the kind Dr. Hendricks-Ferguson has made on me, will leave a mark. She is a remarkable professional and greatly respected, and very loved.

I enjoy channeling my inner Verna. So, you see, she's more than just a nursing educator, a mere mortal. She is a force, the pulse and the endowment deep within me. I owe my career in oncology nursing, and its success, to her. ❧

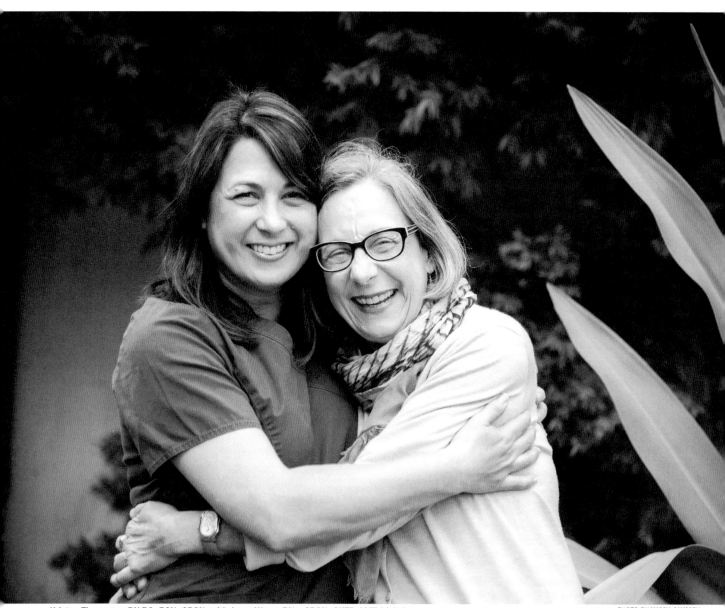

Kristen Thompson, RN-BC, BSN, CPON, with Joyce Wong, RNc, CPON, CHTP, LMT [right]

My Beautiful Princess

KRISTEN THOMPSON, RN-BC, BSN, CPON

[KAPIOLANI MEDICAL CENTER FOR WOMEN AND CHILDREN IN HONOLULU, HAWAII]

WRITTEN BY JOYCE WONG, RNC, CPON, CHTP, LMT

SLEEPING SOUNDLY, 5-year-old Malia moved slowly in her bed, teddy and blanket close to her side. Kristen had come into her room, following her assignment, checking on her patient. Yes, IV intact and chemo running without incident (check). Breathing, pulse and temperature all within normal limits (check). Child's positioned well, good alignment and bed linens clean and orderly (check). Side rails up and call light close (check). It was a routine day for Kristen, who is an excellent and experienced pediatric oncology nurse, but for Malia it was a dream come true.

MALIA OPENED HER EYES wide and said, "Cinderella, is that really you?" Kristen has an attractive face (she is Chinese and German), her light brown-blonde hair tied back loosely this day, and she was wearing a blue scrub top. The light from a nearby window shown on her hair and it glistened. Kristen smiled widely, a sweet, warm smile and said, "Yes, my dear; I am here to care for you with love and all my attention." Malia smiled back and laughed. "Nurse Kristen…You are my Cinderella!"

Kristen is an extraordinary nurse who can be "Cinderella" in one room and go to the next one to hold the hand of a palliative care patient who is taking their last breaths. All this with integrity, warmth, sincerity and excellence skills.

Kristen is a teacher and mentor to the younger generation of oncology nurses, able to tell true and touching stories about her patients, while also teaching the medical aspects of leukemia and other cancers. She gets down to the nitty-gritty with staff, teaching them important points of actual nursing care, including clinical information to make our jobs go more smoothly.

Kristen is an integral member of the team, using good communication with physician, occupational therapists and physical therapists, nutritionists, social workers, child life specialists, psychiatrists and fellow nurses. Patients and families often ask if Kristen could be "their child's nurse."

"Cinderella" moves through her day with a smooth energy flow, giving heart-centered care with an impeccable demeanor. Her scrubs could easily be traded for an elaborate sequenced ball gown!

"Cinderella" also makes annual appearances at the Cancer Camp for children of all ages, and especially one for teens with cancer. She comes incognito in shorts and a T-shirt, but her golden heart abides. She acts as counselor to teens with issues of body image, loss, school and peer problems and fears and worries. This teen camp allows for expression to professionals and an opportunity to grow and mature with them, as well as fellow survivors. Kristen is a strong counselor and role model.

TEACHING MOMENT:

Kristen is a teacher and mentor to the younger generation of oncology nurses, able to tell true and touching stories about her patients, while also teaching the medical aspects of leukemia and other cancers.

Kristen is truly a "Cinderella" of pediatric oncology nursing, as she is very humble and open but professional and conservative in her ways. She would quietly laugh and tell the story about Malia but is one who rather been doing her work, instead of in the limelight. But beware, when you would least expect it, a whole hallway of admirers could come down upon Kristen, offering a glass slipper to the one who is the true "Princess Cinderella" of pediatric oncology nursing. Ah, yes. It fits!

Thank you, Kristen, for this and all of the "Cinderella Moments" you have brought to patients at Kapiolani Medical Center for Women and Children! ❧

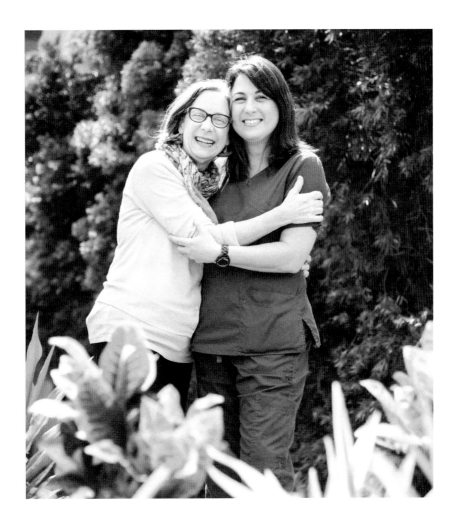

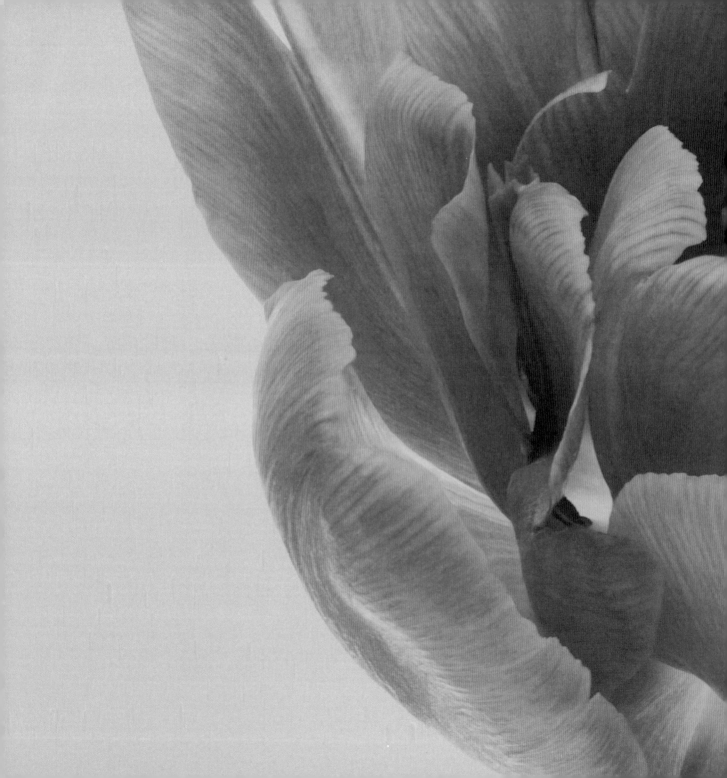

CHAPTER 3
For a Loved One

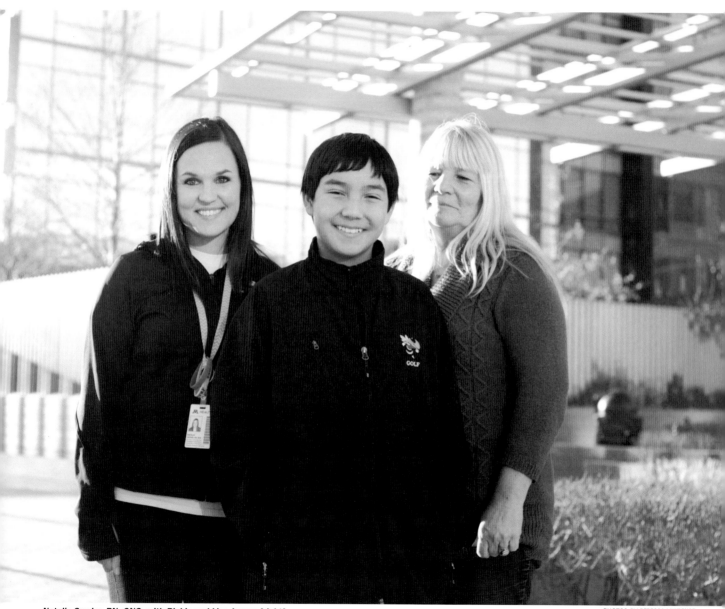

Natalie Snyder, RN, ONC, with Richie and Lisa Jenson [right]

The Best Thing for an 11-Year-Old Boy's Cancer: His Amazing Nurse!

NATALIE SNYDER, RN, ONC

[UNIVERSITY OF MINNESOTA AMPLATZ CHILDREN'S HOSPITAL IN MINNEAPOLIS, MINNESOTA]

WRITTEN BY LISA JENSON

MY SON RICHIE was diagnosed with Ewing's sarcoma in February 2013. Needless to say, we were all terrified at the diagnosis. Richie has always had a fear of "shots," so much so that I wouldn't tell him if he had an upcoming appointment for his immunizations with his doctor for fear he wouldn't sleep at all the night before the appointment.

IN THE 10 DAYS following his initial diagnosis, he had three surgeries, three biopsies and a power port placement. Three days after the power port was placed, he had a PET scan. It was his very first port access. It went terribly wrong. There was still gauze over his port from the placement surgery, and no one had told us about the numbing cream that was to be applied 15 minutes prior to access to numb the area on his chest where they were going to poke him with two needles.

There was glue that was applied during the placement of the port to seal up the incision. As the PET scan nurse took off the gauze bandage, it was adhered to the glue on the incision. She had to gain access to his port, so she pulled it off all the while he was screaming and crying in pain. There was no time to wait for the numbing cream to work, she said, as their schedule for the PET scanner was booked. So she accessed his port that was extremely sore already amidst his screams and my tears.

He said he never wanted anyone to access his port again. Richie was scheduled to start his three months of chemotherapy in five days. When we got to the hospital for the first round of chemo, he was scared to death about anyone even touching his port. I was praying that Richie would have a better experience this time accessing his port than the first time; I knew there would be so many more accesses throughout the next nine

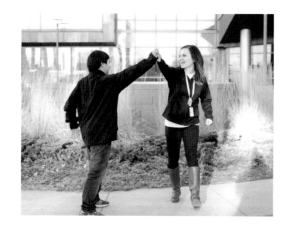

months of his treatment.

We both had tears in our eyes as the most incredible nurse walked into the room; it was Natalie. She has a gentle spirit and a calming, comforting way about her. Natalie told Richie everything was going to be all right and that she would be his nurse today and would be accessing his port.

He was very nervous, and I could see his hands trembling as she told him to hop up on the bed. She told him this shouldn't hurt and that he should think about a happy place. I had already put the numbing cream on this time. He hopped up on the bed; he held my hand and he went to his "happy place." In no time, Natalie

TEACHING MOMENT:

For someone to be so genuinely caring and compassionate with her patients, and continue to do so even after suffering losses, is truly inspiring to me.

accessed his port. He didn't even feel it!

From that moment on, his whole attitude changed about going to the hospital and getting all his treatments. Richie quickly named Natalie as his favorite nurse and requested her every time we went to the hospital. She has great compassion for all her little patients; she treats them with empathy and love.

As the months of treatment wore on, I came to see what an incredibly hard job it was to be a pediatric oncology nurse. Some of the little patients Natalie had taken care of didn't make it. I could sense this when I entered the floor; it was never spoken, but I could just feel the sadness around me. For someone to be so genuinely caring and compassionate with her patients, and continue to be so even after suffering losses, is truly inspiring to me.

Natalie gave Richie a sense of hope and happiness every time he saw her. Natalie even came up with the idea of making a video of the children on Unit 5 to "Brave" by Sara Bareilles. She spent hours and hours of her free time on it last summer while she was in the midst of planning her own wedding.

The video went viral on YouTube and has over a million views. Natalie was portraying how brave the children were on Unit 5, but I think the nurses, especially Natalie, are just as brave. Natalie is brave by giving her love and compassion to the children, all the while knowing she will face heartbreak when one of them doesn't make it.

Richie was one of the patients in this video, and just being in it has changed his outlook on life. Richie is no longer afraid of anything, he says; he will spend his life being brave just like the video.

Richie is, at present, cancer-free, and a better individual because of the extraordinary care and compassion of Natalie Snyder. She not only taught him a lot about cancer, but she taught him so much more about life and compassion.

Still today, whenever we go to a clinic visit, we always have to go up to the fifth floor of the hospital and see if Natalie is working. Richie loves her so much. If she is working, he won't leave the hospital without giving her a hug and seeing how she is doing. Natalie Snyder not only gave my son her expertise as a great pediatric oncology nurse, but she gave her love, compassion, hope and empathy to him, which I will be eternally grateful for. ❧

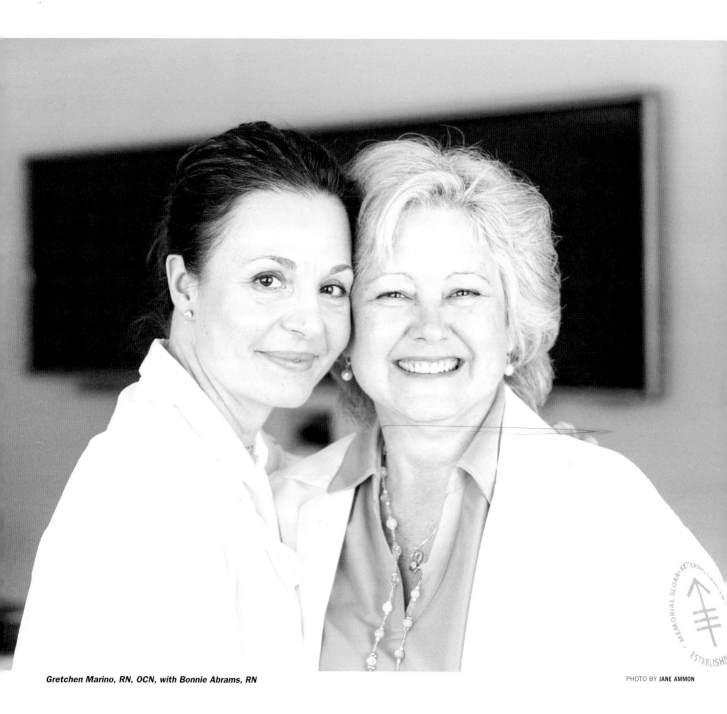

Gretchen Marino, RN, OCN, with Bonnie Abrams, RN

Over and Above: A Nurse Shows Her Wings

GRETCHEN MARINO, RN, OCN

[MEMORIAL SLOAN KETTERING CANCER CENTER IN NEW YORK, NEW YORK]

WRITTEN BY BONNIE ABRAMS, RN

MY NAME IS BONNIE ABRAMS. I have been a nurse for more than 30 years. I work with cancer patients every day at Memorial Sloan Kettering Cancer Center, and I love what I do. But, this is not my story; this is the story of a nurse who stood next to me during a terrible storm in my life. She held my hand and guided me through the darkness, with her skills and expertise, down a road I never thought I would travel. Her name is Gretchen Marino.

EVERY SO OFTEN, no matter how good we are as nurses at fending off what comes our way, life throws us a curve ball. It can have long-reaching and everlasting effects on a person and his or her family. It can change us forever. Luckily for me, when this occurred in my life, Gretchen was there to catch me and help guide me through the storm.

It was about four years ago that my husband woke up one Saturday morning and told me he had a lump in his throat that wouldn't go away. We had season tickets to the Yankees that year and a game that day. I sat next to him in the stadium, looking at him, and I knew in the pit of my stomach that something was very wrong.

We spent the next couple weeks waiting for test results. The days were long and torturous. Sleep came in short spurts. Both of us could feel the anxiety of the unknown. Finally, as I sat at my desk at work, head in hand, the doctor who had received Jeff's test results walked around the corner. Jeff had stage 4 esophageal cancer, a type of cancer that is usually both aggressive and deadly. We talked awhile and then she told me,

"Gretchen will be in touch with you today."

In an instant, my relationship with Gretchen changed from a nursing colleague to a patient's wife in her care. Everything I knew about this disease frightened me beyond belief. How would Jeff get through this? How would I get through this?

After speaking with Gretchen that afternoon, I knew she would always be there for us. And she was. She held my hand when I cried, answered my questions (some I didn't realize I had), and used her expert knowledge and experience to help us navigate through the cancer web.

TEACHING MOMENT:

When Jeff needed to talk about his feelings and thoughts, he would often reach out to her. She would always listen and gently answer him openly and honestly.

Gretchen found me hope when I felt hopeless. She knew how to turn a tear into a smile with her tender, caring compassion and understanding. She would reach out to me with a hug or a kind word during the more difficult times.

As my husband's disease progressed, Gretchen always anticipated our needs. She helped prepare us emotionally and supported us through the transition into hospice care. Throughout my husband's disease, Gretchen would encourage us to live for the day and be grateful for all the moments we had together. She had the ability to make us feel as though we were her first and only priority. Gretchen provided us with the compassion and support that we needed so we never felt alone.

Jeff lived for two years. He weathered well the chemotherapy, radiation and stents he had placed in his throat. He always believed he was going to beat his disease. He lived, as many cancer patients do, every day to the fullest. He had no pain and very few "down days." Gretchen was his hero. When Jeff needed to talk about his feelings and thoughts, he would often reach out to her. She would always listen and gently answer him openly and honestly. Gretchen would never side-step any question. Answering the difficult questions helped Jeff battle his denial and gave him the courage to take and keep control of his life.

Losing my husband was the single most difficult journey in my life. It was Gretchen who lit the path, gave me insight, gave me strength when I was crumbling and never let me falter. Gretchen epitomizes what this award symbolizes, and as a coworker and "the patient's family," I will always be one of her biggest fans. Life may have thrown me a curve ball, but I was able to hit it out of the park because of Gretchen. ❧

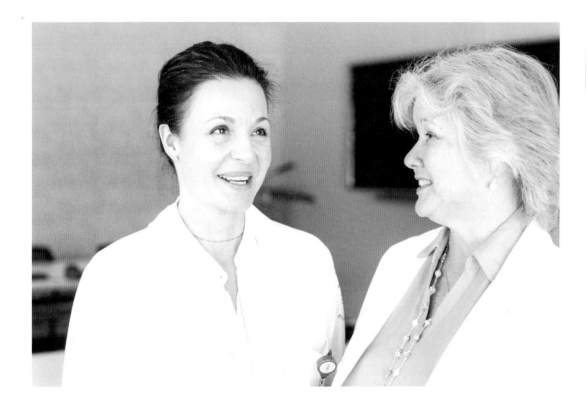

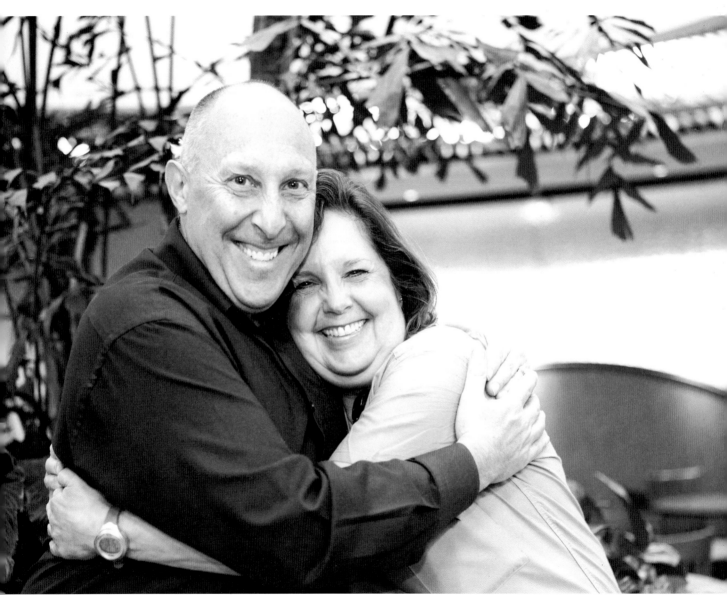

Andy Himes with Wendy Lien, RN [right]

Connecting with the Heart

WENDY LIEN, RN [SKY RIDGE MEDICAL CENTER IN LONE TREE, COLORADO]

WRITTEN BY ANDY HIMES

MY WIFE passed away on Feb. 2, 2014, from a six-year battle with cancer. It is my honor to nominate one angel in particular who, in the end, became much more than a nurse to my wife. Her name is Wendy and she works in the interventional radiology department at Sky Ridge Medical Center.

IN EARLY 2013, my wife Rosa developed a condition called pleural effusion due to her metastatic breast cancer on both sides of her lungs. She began going to the interventional radiology department on a regular basis to have fluid drained. That is where she met Wendy. It didn't take long before they developed a very special friendship and connection.

My wife was always very cheerful and upbeat. She had a very infectious smile and the sweetest personality. She was everyone's favorite patient because she never complained and always seemed to be happy to the point of cracking jokes here and there.

When Rosa was scheduled for an appointment, it was not unusual for several nurses, including Wendy, to greet her and give her a big hug welcoming her. Consequently, going to Sky Ridge Medical Center became something she looked forward to because of all the kindness she received from everyone!

Wendy took a special interest in Rosa. She not only assisted in the procedures to drain fluid, but she would also visit her over in oncology while she was undergoing chemotherapy. Wendy would simply sit and visit with Rosa, and it was just a special time for both of them as they got to know each other. When Rosa was hospitalized for the last time in January, Wendy came up to her room often to visit her and even help answer questions we may have had with all the different doctors.

Rosa told me often how much she loved Wendy and wanted to schedule time outside of the hospital to get together, perhaps for dinner. We never got that chance, unfortunately.

Wendy was always available for phone calls. She not only talked with Rosa if she was having an issue at home, but she was always available to me when I had questions and she often helped coordinate appointments between her department and oncology. Rosa's condition became particularly complex as she eventually was unable to have any more fluid drained because of how thick it had become. Wendy helped us understand what was going on.

TEACHING MOMENT:

I am nominating Wendy because she not only demonstrated extraordinary expertise and competence, she also went way above and beyond in sharing her heart, friendship and wonderful compassion.

One evening, Rosa asked the sweetest question to me. It still brings tears to my eyes when I think about it. Rosa asked me how she would go about asking Wendy if she would be her best friend!

At Rosa's service on Feb. 15, I played an audio clip from a visit she had with her oncologist a couple of months prior. It was Rosa at her very best. The conversation was about what to do if fluid started building up again, and Rosa was very clear on what to do: "Wendy." She went on to joke about all the hugs she got when she went over there, and even her oncologist joked about her being in the frequent flyer club! It was a cute conversation, and I treasure it.

There is so much sadness surrounding my wife's illness and death. The journey of cancer is a very long, gut-wrenching and all-too-often painful journey. But it is also a journey of love. My wife and I shared so much love during those six years. We never stopped traveling, and we never stopped fighting this dreaded disease. We were an incredible team. Along the way, we also met countless angels of mercy. From doctors to

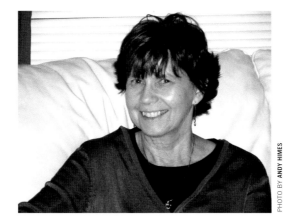

Rosa Himes

friends, from medical providers to all the incredible nurses—and to Wendy. It is those memories and people like Wendy who will always remain instrumental in my own healing journey.

I am nominating Wendy because she not only demonstrated extraordinary expertise and competence, she also went way above and beyond in sharing her heart, friendship and wonderful compassion. I think this part of medicine gets lost in this day and age of science and technology. Cancer is a dreaded disease that devastates the body, but it is also equally devastating emotionally. Wendy is a rare individual who understands healing is not just about a procedure. It is also about connecting with the heart. ❧

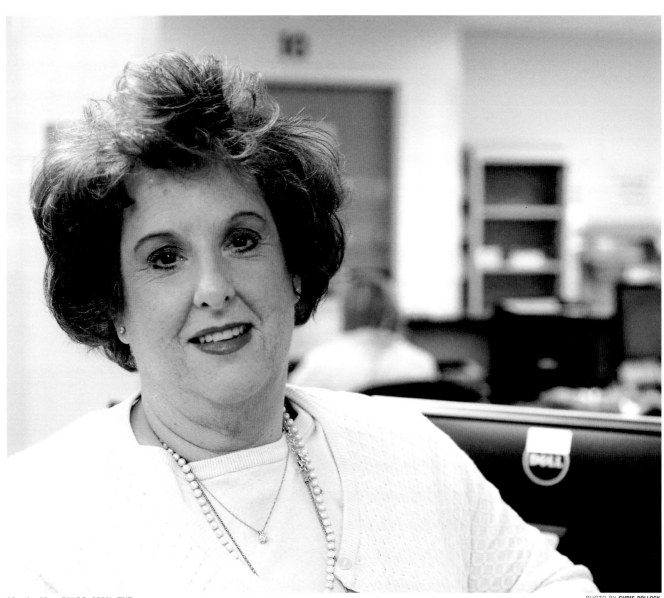

Martha May, RN-CS, MSN, FNP

A Comforting Soul

MARTHA MAY, RN-CS, MSN, FNP [ST. JUDE CHILDREN'S RESEARCH HOSPITAL IN MEMPHIS, TENNESSEE]

WRITTEN BY SHELBY SONORA

IT SEEMS IMPOSSIBLE to me to put into words just how special St. Jude Children's Research Hospital nurse practitioner Martha May is to my family. At a time when our world was completely turned upside down and became chaotic, she brought a genuine love and caring to that world.

I WILL NEVER FORGET my little girl, Yesenia, being in isolation for months, and the whole world of leukemia was completely foreign to us. We had so many questions. But something as simple as the sound of shoes clinking on the floors of the hallways of St. Jude became one of the most comforting sounds to me and my daughter.

Yesenia's treatment for her leukemia involved several types of procedures. These appointments always scared me and made me feel very nervous. Miss Martha, our special nurse, did everything she could to ease my worries by performing these procedures herself. Martha wore these little shoes that would "clink" as she walked down the hall. Hearing that clink would bring me peace and calmness because I knew that she was coming to talk to us and explain just exactly what was going on. She always made us feel comfortable and explained what to expect next.

She would tell me, "I'll take good care of her. I'll find y'all at the picture." I would kiss my little girl on the cheek and walk down the hall to the "Mickey and Minnie" picture and wait. Time almost seemed to stop. I know that these procedures only took a few minutes to complete, but it always felt so much longer.

Then I would hear the clink. Oh, that calming clink. I could breathe again. Martha would always turn the corner of the hallway with a big smile on her face, letting us know that everything was OK. Every time we saw her, we knew just how lucky and blessed we were to have her as our nurse and our friend.

Martha always has such a positive attitude. Her smile and bubbly personality are contagious and a joy to be around. She brought warmth and comfort to our world when we needed it the most. She is consistent, kind and full of joy.

She listens to you, even when you are not speaking. Martha was so patient with our endless questions and concerns. She and my daughter had a special relationship that grew and blossomed. Yesenia would go home and practice songs that she wanted to sing for Martha. Martha's reactions to the songs made Yesenia feel like she was on cloud nine. Our trips to St. Jude felt so familiar, so comfortable, like Yesenia was home.

Miss Martha is our beautiful angel. I can't tell her enough how much I'm so grateful for her and the work she does. She puts so much effort into her work and it shows. Because of that, my daughter has been given a second chance at life. Martha is obedient to God's calling, to be His hands and feet. Jesus said in Matthew 25:35-40:

"For I was hungry and you gave me something to eat, I was thirsty and you gave me something to drink, I was a stranger and you invited me in. I needed clothes and you clothed me, I was sick and you looked after me, I was in prison and you came to visit me. Then the righteous will answer him, 'Lord, when did we see you hungry and feed you, or thirsty and give you something to drink? When did we see you a stranger and invite you in, or needing clothes and clothe you? When did we see you sick or in prison and go to visit you?' The King will reply, 'Truly I tell you, whatever you did for one of the least of these brothers of mine, you did for me.'

The founder of modern nursing, Florence Nightingale, wrote the following, and I feel like it fits appropriately to Miss Martha:

"Nursing is an art, and if it is to be made an art, it requires an exclusive devotion, as hard a preparation, as any painter's or sculptor's work; for what is the having to do with dead canvas or dead marble, compared with having to do with the living body, the temple of God's spirit? It is one of the Fine Arts; I had almost said, the finest of Fine Arts." ❧

Lucy's Eyes

LUCY HERTEL, RN, BSN, OCN

[WASHINGTON UNIVERSITY IN ST. LOUIS, SCHOOL OF MEDICINE, IN ST. LOUIS MISSOURI]

WRITTEN BY SUE PECK

LUCY is an oncology nurse with very special eyes. The light in Lucy's eyes is extraordinary. The beholder is held captive.

IT IS A DEEP HURT for the pain of the patient. It reflects her deep intense feeling to help. To be able to share the suffering of a cancer patient is a gift given to Lucy. Best of all, she is willing to share this gift. My sister is a cancer patient. I am her caregiver.

Lucy's eyes give my sister and me compassion, understanding, thoughtfulness, fire for life, laughter, joy, help and determination. What affects my sister ... affects her!

My name is Sue. My sister's name is Betty. I was with her when she was given the cancer diagnosis. I recall thinking that I must stay strong for her. However, I was lost, sad, confused and despondent. I thought it would be easier to die than to give her up.

I am 78 years old. She is 80. We have raised our families and shared many wonderful days. I just could not imagine a life without her. She is my confidant, my traveling companion and my keeper of secrets. What would I do?

In despair, I looked up into Lucy's eyes. The light I saw there radiated compassion. Without speaking, she transferred her understanding of my pain. The thoughtfulness in her eyes showed that she knew what I was feeling. It was powerful enough to say, without a word, "I will help you take care of your sister."

Imagine the wave of relief that came flowing into my soul. There, in the doctor's office, I handed Lucy my heart. And in an unspoken whisper said, "Thank you." Without a doubt, the light in Lucy's eyes had conveyed the message that she was able to understand the feelings of another. She had projected the courage that was so desperately needed. I had received a marvelous gift.

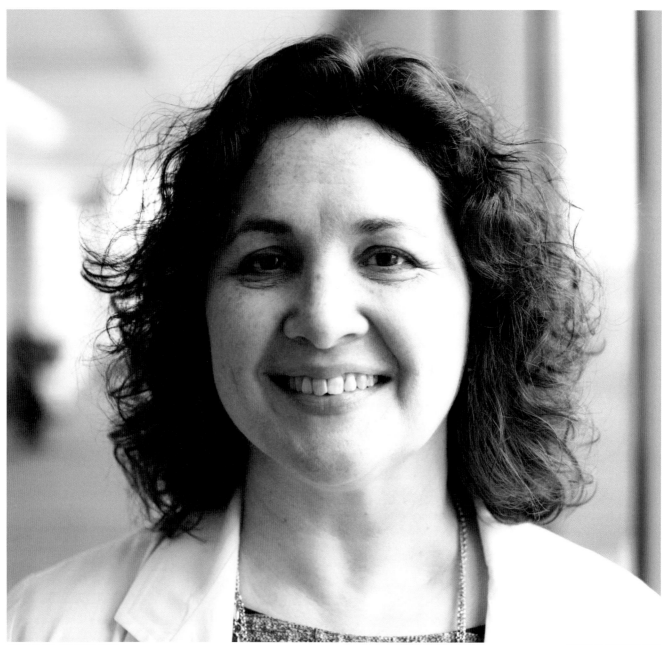

Lucy Hertel, RN, BSN, OCN

There is fire in Lucy's eyes when she speaks earnestly to her patients. There are no promises of miracles. She tells no lies. She goes directly to the point and is painfully honest. The patient wants to hear something good and positive. Lucy's response is, "We are ready to try a new approach. The doctor and I will do everything possible to help you." Assurance that all is being done is what one needs. Lucy, with fire in her eyes, tells you that and you believe her.

Lucy's eyes sparkle with laughter. Her eyes twinkle with pleasure as the bubbling laughter escapes. Whether it is a feather in a cap that covers a bald head or a funny sound a patient makes while being stuck with a needle, she can laugh. It is Lucy's responsibility to make sure the patient and caregiver are aware of dates of treatments, required blood tests and doctor's appointments.

She creates a monthly calendar with all the necessary information. She giggles as she marks the dates and makes happy comments such as, "We will sure be happy to see you in three weeks." Her eyes glow with a feeling of joy that relays that there is much to look forward to at our next visit.

For a
Loved One

TEACHING MOMENT:

Assurance that all is being done is what one needs. Lucy, with fire in her eyes, tells you that and you believe her.

Lucy's eyes can cry with no tears. She does not avoid the pain or the sadness. She faces them with eyes so full of tears that it is impossible to know how she contains them. The joy of laughter is gone, the fire of expectations disappears and the compassion for pain is intensified. She strangles the sobs with a long deep breath. She needs extra strength to deal with both the patient and the caregiver. She is determined to give that care without tears. This wonderful nurse displays an inner core that is immeasurable by human standards. It is impossible to explain.

Lucy's eyes can accept. Lucy's eyes become darker, calmer and project that it is no longer a choice of acceptance or rejection. She does not glance away. She faces the inevitable head on. The absolute peaceful realization of life and death shines through her eyes like a beacon from a lighthouse. She offers a course to follow to the end. An awareness of her determination to share the hardest part is put forth by the kindness in her eyes.

Avoiding reality is not her style. She confronts truth with eyes that do not blink. Lucy, with her medical knowledge, does not hide from the truth. Through her eyes, she gives the patient the courage to accept the outcome. Lucy is strong and she makes the patient strong.

Lucy inspires confidence in the doctor. She is full of assurance in the other members of the staff and relates great stories about the work they do. She understands that the patient is struggling to cope. Her eyes smile with the serenity of hope and inspiration.

What wonderful gifts from an extraordinary oncology nurse. These gifts cannot be purchased. They cannot be earned. They must come through the light in Lucy's eyes! ❧

CHAPTER 4
Life & Laughter

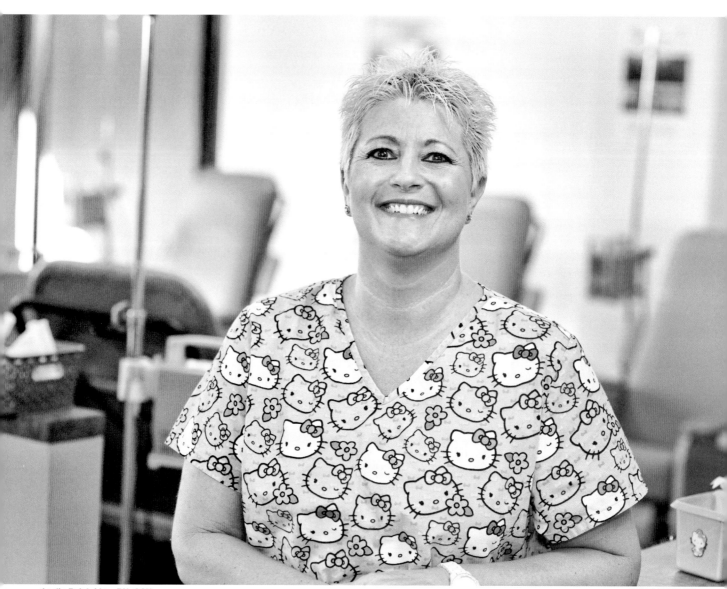

Leslie Bainbridge, RN, OCN

My Encourager

LESLIE BAINBRIDGE, RN, OCN [ARIZONA ONCOLOGY IN PHOENIX, ARIZONA]

WRITTEN BY JOYCE BOWERS

"WHO CAN TURN THE WORLD ON WITH HER SMILE?" Not Mary Tyler Moore, but instead my oncology nurse, Leslie Bainbridge of Arizona Oncology. My first introduction to Leslie was about 30 days after a grueling four-hour debulking surgery for stage 3c primary peritoneal carcinoma.

I WAS FEELING EXTREMELY VULNERABLE and still a bit confused when I first met Leslie, who was to be my chemotherapy nurse. She would be the person I would see weekly to mix and administer all of my chemotherapy medications. The only thing about that first meeting I remember through the haze is asking Leslie if she thought she could handle my case. Without pausing, she very confidently explained to me that she would take extremely good care of me and that we were on this journey together. I remember her speaking to me as though I were an old friend. Her eyes were warm and her smile was ever present as she explained how the medications would work and that I could definitely "do this" and get through these treatments.

Another time I remember laughing with her was when I first spied the chemo room. It was decked out with positive words on posters and little signs. There were many "Girl Power" inspiring words in every nook and cranny of that room. Another time I came into the chemo room and Leslie had redecorated it to look as though we were at the islands. There were leis and silk flowers draped everywhere. She wanted her chemo receivers to feel as though we were somewhere else during our four- to six-hour chemo treatments. Leslie Bainbridge became my sparkling cheerleader and never-ending encourager.

Who really wants to keep a chemotherapy appointment anyway? I found that during the first four months, and even now as I am in my first recurrence, my answer to that question is an emphatic *me*. Seeing

Leslie every week was where I would discover a wealth of information, as well as uncover laughter and the strength to keep going with my treatments. Leslie could even make a comedy act out of checking my birthday against what my medications read: "Oh, it hasn't changed since the last time you were here, good deal!"

To be embraced with a hug and a huge smile and Leslie's happy attitude can turn an ordinary day into an extraordinary day. She always makes me feel as though I am an integral part of her day and not just another patient on her list to care for. She is totally familiar with my case, and if I have a question she can't answer, she will research it to find the best solution. This was true when a pharmacist expressed concern about a chemotherapy medication reacting to one of my regular daily medications. Leslie found a specialist who solved the dilemma for us, thus easing a very stressful situation for me. Leslie never gives up, but instead uses many resources to enhance the care she gives to me. This teamwork makes me want to fight and continue on to get rid of this cancer. I don't want to let Leslie down; she gives me her all and the least I can do is keep fighting in return. She is my inspiration to do just that.

TEACHING MOMENT:

Seeing Leslie every week was where I would discover a wealth of information, as well as uncover laughter and the strength to keep going with my treatments.

I have personally observed Leslie dealing compassionately with a young woman receiving end-of-life care. I watched as this woman was guided through the door of the chemo room. Leslie's face lit up calling to her like an old friend. After hugs and laughter, I saw as Leslie's skilled hands virtually flew while meeting needs as she calmed the young woman with a warm blanket and soothing and encouraging words. She makes all of us calmer, while her kind words of cheer and praise enable us to feel like conquerors.

Leslie compels me to believe I am a peer when I am with her and not just another cancer patient fighting for her life. While she administers the medications, she continually expresses hope that what she is giving to me might just be the ticket to kill this roguish cancer. I always perceive that Leslie is just as invested in my healing as I am.

What a delight it is to receive a personal email from Leslie, whether it is simply asking how I am doing or to give advice on foods that will make me feel better or help improve my low protein or potassium levels. Reading her words, I can almost see her effervescent personality linking healing and humor with caring. Her words shout out to me that she is on my side and she is cheering me on to a state of wellness.

When I am feeling insecure about where I stand in actively fighting this first recurrence of primary peritoneal carcinoma, it helps immeasurably to understand that Leslie has dealt with these recurrences before. She knows the different protocols that are available and can expertly explain each of them to me as well as their possible side effects. I truly appreciate that she keeps a trained eye on me and can spot anything potentially going wrong. I do not feel alone; I feel supported by Leslie in every step I take.

To sum up my relationship with my oncology nurse Leslie Bainbridge, I am happy to include the following: Leslie is passionate about seeing cancer eradicated in each of her patients. She grasps the banner of encouragement and gently drapes it over the shoulders of each chemotherapy recipient she comes in contact with. She is adamant that a sense of normalcy while living with cancer is a healthy and beneficial way to live. Leslie demonstrates this by making me feel like a welcome friend as I enter her domain and never like a cancer patient. She has added hope and joy to my life.

I could not even imagine traveling this journey without her. ✖

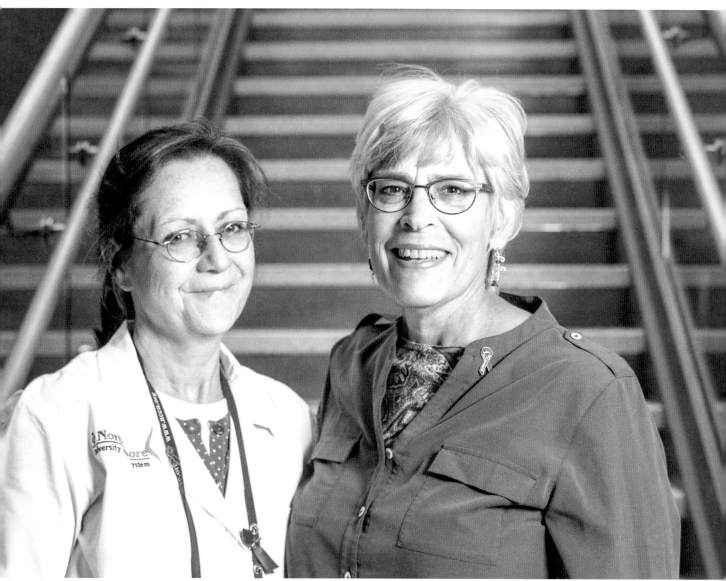

Margaret Whalen, RN, BSN, with Susan Howard [right]

My Kind of Nurse

MARGARET WHALEN, RN, BSN [NORTHSHORE UNIVERSITY HEALTHSYSTEM IN EVANSTON, ILLINOIS]

WRITTEN BY SUSAN HOWARD

MARGARET WHALEN is my kind of nurse! Margaret Whalen exemplifies all of the critically important qualities an oncology nurse must possess to provide excellent care to her patients. Let me tell you my "Margaret Story." It begins on April 1, 2013, when, after several weeks of symptoms, I was diagnosed with inoperable stage 3 pancreatic cancer. The physicians who provided the diagnosis told me to go ahead with my planned scuba diving vacation to Grand Cayman. Armed with steroids, enzymes and other meds, I was able to get to the Caribbean.

FOR THE NEXT WEEK I cried often, thinking maybe it was the last I would see of that gorgeous blue water. I managed to do a few dives and filled my mask with many tears. The time away in the Caribbean turned out to be a godsend, completely unrelated to diving and blue water. It provided the time needed to reflect on what I wanted in cancer treatment.

Soon after our return, in a twist of fate, we were set up to see an oncologist, Dr. Marsh. He walked in smiling, pulled up an exam stool and said he was saving the "throne" at the computer for Margaret, his nurse. He said she got the throne because that was where the important work got done. This seemed to be a reverential recommendation from a doctor who recognized Margaret's importance to him and his patients.

My husband and I had a two-hour appointment that day—two hours of talking about diagnosis, information about clinical trials, review of my proposed treatment plan, education about the chemotherapy I would take, how they would follow my progress and response to treatment and even an overview of future treatment and surgery based on my response to treatment.

Dr. Marsh eventually left us in Margaret's capable hands. Together we sat comfortably until all of our questions were answered, the plan firm in our minds and my first treatment set up there in order to expedite treatment, with future treatments set up at another hospital that was more convenient for us.

Margaret talked with us as a patient-provider team. Our goal was to reduce tumor mass and make the tumor operable, which was my only chance for a cure. Wow!

TEACHING MOMENT:

Every time I had chemotherapy, Margaret was around to answer questions that I had or that the nurses had about me, or maybe to just poke her head in and allay my fears in her calm, reassuring way.

Both she and Dr. Marsh made us feel like we could beat this nasty disease. Margaret walked us out of the office and downstairs to the door. She smiled and said, "Someday we will be talking about this meeting." I felt at home with her. She was just like my nurse friends who are excellent nurses on all counts.

All the way home, my husband and I talked about how different a mood and feeling we got from this visit. We were buoyed, and hope was restored. Who could be smiling with a diagnosis of pancreatic cancer? We were! And we were anxious to start.

On the first day of chemotherapy, Margaret had also prearranged for the rest of the team to see me: the social worker, oncology dietitian/nutritionist and pharmacist. Everything was in place. And every time I had chemotherapy, Margaret was around to answer questions that I had or that the nurses had about me, or maybe to just poke her head in and allay my fears in her calm, reassuring way.

She always seemed calm, but I learned, on a moment's notice, she would make an assessment and spring into action. One day while I was having chemo, she stopped by to check on me. Carefully questioning me, she determined I was having a side effect that had started soon after my chemo nurse had stepped out of the room. She quietly said she would be right back. The next thing I knew, the rapid response team of my chemo nurse, a second nurse and the pharmacist were there in a flash, evaluated my chemo response and took care of me. No muss, no fuss, just Margaret's business as usual.

Margaret never expected my 36 years of nursing experience to be a substitute for the information she provided for me, her patient. When I had questions about how I felt or my medications that I felt just couldn't wait until my next visit, she was always readily responsive that day by phone, despite her long hours and many patients.

It is now almost one year to the day that I started feeling sick. I have been through chemo, radiation therapy with chemo, a long Whipple surgery and more chemo. Margaret was there through it all. I am happy to say it has been a year because I am a one-year survivor of pancreatic cancer.

This chapter of my "Margaret Story" ends. I plan to be a long-term survivor, and I know Margaret will walk in survival with me, making future chapters in the story possible.

Margaret Whalen has and will continue to epitomize for me what a nurse should be: competent, caring, compassionate, calm and calming, conscientious, and all with a sense of humor. She is my kind of nurse, and I am so happy and fortunate that she is mine! ❧

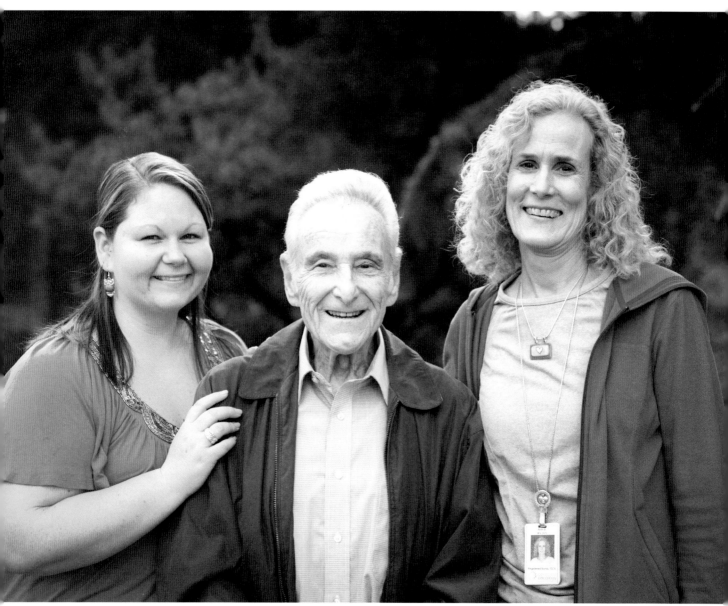

Samantha Itkin with her grandfather, Louis, and Ann E. Grotz, RN, OCN [right]

Our Nurse IS the Best Medicine

ANN E. GROTZ, RN, OCN [COMPASS ONCOLOGY IN PORTLAND, OREGON]

WRITTEN BY SAMANTHA ITKIN

I WOULD LIKE TO NOMINATE one of our current nurses, the extraordinary Ann E. Grotz, a registered nurse at Compass Oncology, for this year's award. She is a compassionate, extremely helpful and expert oncology nurse, and I hope to express this to you throughout this essay. Ann deserves the Extraordinary Healer Award for Oncology Nursing because of the high level of care and support she provides for my 86-year-old grandfather who is fighting colon cancer for the second time within the past year.

IN EARLY 2013, my grandfather was diagnosed with colon cancer. After having his surgery and then taking time to recuperate, he started his chemotherapy treatment at Compass Oncology East in Portland, Oregon, a short time later. As many can imagine, and others know, this process is tremendously stressful on not only the patient, but the caregiver as well. The first time we arrived at the clinic we met several helpful and caring nurses. Though many, if not all, of the nurses at this location go above and beyond their requirements to make my grandfather and other patients feel at ease, Ann is the one that really has been accommodating and compassionate the most.

After my grandfather was in remission for a short two months, we returned to the clinic, but became worried when we didn't see Ann during the first couple of visits. We were so thankful when she returned from her time off because we couldn't imagine going through this without her kindness, smile and laughter.

Below are some examples that demonstrate why Ann should be the winner of this year's award.

She is always willing to find out the answer to my grandfather's random questions. On our last visit he wanted to know the meaning of some abbreviations on his blood work. Ann overheard my grandfather asking me, and within a few minutes, she brought over a printout to help him, explaining the abbreviations and advising him that there would be a quiz on it at next week's visit. This made him smile, and when he smiles, that makes me smile.

She sure does adapt to his silly sense of humor and makes our visits easier. During this same visit, I made a comment to my grandfather that he didn't drink enough water. Before he could tell me he knew what to do, Ann stepped in and backed me, told him to drink more water because he needed it. I am so thankful for her willingness to help me as a caregiver in addition to helping my grandfather as the patient.

A few visits before that my grandfather was concerned about his nose that consistently drips. Ann quickly responded that it could be a side effect of one of the chemotherapy drugs he is taking. Another time, my grandfather was worried about me accidently taking a bite of his food after he had eaten off of it and that I might be in danger. Ann smiled and let him know I wasn't going to be hurt by this, but that we should not make this a habit. Ann always makes time to give my grandfather the information he wants to know.

It is amazing how she handles all the patients with their different personalities. As for my grandfather, he is one with a good sense of humor. Each visit he asks her for a cold beer instead of his chemotherapy, and Ann always has a quick-witted response with a sneering smile that makes us both laugh. Another time I witnessed her helping another elderly patient who clearly didn't want to be there. Ann changed her approach from the joking entertaining self to a concerned, charismatic caregiver. This is just a brief example of how Ann changes her nursing style to meet all of her patients.

When my grandfather goes in to have his chemotherapy pump removed, he always hopes to get "Annie," as she is the swift and best at removing the tape that holds the Infusystem to his port. He tells her that she should open up a shop called the Super Express Swift Shaving Chest Parlor. As usual, she responds with a smile and says, "Oh yes, right!" It's conversations like this that really set Ann apart from other nurses.

My grandfather also wanted me to mention that Ann wears some crazy shoes that catch many of the

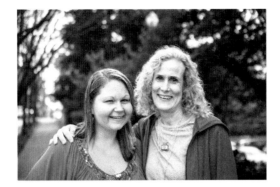

patient's attention and wonders where she gets them. Each visit, I remind him that they are her Danskos, which are comfortable nurse shoes. He hopes she gets another pair after she wins this award that she truly deserves because of her hard work, dedication and support that she has provided him through this last challenging year.

It is hard to wrap up all the reasons why Ann should be this year's winner in a short essay because she is truly extraordinary and has brought many smiles, joy and happiness to my grandfather and me, as well as other patients we have met. Though there are many nurses we have met and not met, Ann stands out to my grandfather and me as a supporter on many different levels. She has made a huge impact for us. Her continued inspiration, compassion, helpfulness and support sets her apart and has made this journey of my grandfather's smoother for both him and myself. When watching Ann, you can definitely see that she loves her job and patients, especially knowing she drives over an hour each way to work to care for others.

This is our amazing Ann! I hope you now can agree that she sure is a remarkably extraordinary healer and the best around! ❧

She Gives Me Courage

SUSANNE C. BENTHIN, RN-BSN, OCN [COLUMBIA MEMORIAL HOSPITAL IN ASTORIA, OREGON]

WRITTEN BY MARGARET PATTERSON

MY FAVORITE NURSE, Susanne, is a model in courage and persistence. Good thing, because I am on the fifth year of treatment for breast cancer after developing stage 4 cancer. When I first met Susanne, I already had two surgeries, two recurrences, needle trauma and was very anxious about continuing treatment at all.

SHE WAS SO GOOD WITH ME, and from the first day, talked me through whatever process I had to undergo using guided imagery and reassurance. That first day, she turned my chair away from the busy infusion room, faced me toward a fountain and then asked me where I wanted to go scuba diving and made up an underwater fantasy to get my mind elsewhere while she deftly did her work. It was nothing short of amazing, considering what I had been through. On a previous blood draw, I had walked out (without getting the blood) after seven failed attempts by three different people. From then on, I called Susanne "the vein whisperer."

Over the past five years, I have had blood draws almost every month, along with multiple shots in the belly and… um… elsewhere. I got to the point where if Susanne was unavailable when I arrived, I would simply reschedule for another day and go home! Once, she even arranged to come down to the MRI department to make sure that I had a smooth time with the IV insertion for the contrast dye. She was instrumental in my deciding to get a port, which I had been afraid of, and then when the port also proved painful, she came up with a new protocol for accessing it, using specially arranged equipment (a SafeStep Huber Needle) and techniques to lessen the pain.

Recently, my oncologist moved his practice to another city, and when I told the new nurses about how Susanne accessed my port, they said they didn't do that there. I now have all my blood work orders sent to

Columbia Memorial instead, so I can continue with Susanne. It's that important to me.

She is innovative and caring, and very thoughtful. She always remembers whatever I tell her about my life and family, hopes and fears, and inquires about them at each visit. She arranges hospital services of Reiki treatment, pet therapy and massage treatments for me. She also has experience as a hospice nurse, so she's not afraid to talk with me about death and dying when that's what is on my mind. It's really amazing that I've come this far, outliving my original prognosis by double now, and how much a part of my journey Susanne has been.

My appointments with her have become comforting visits with a dear friend. We discuss our lives, children, parents, share diet and exercise tips, and tell each other of our travels. Once, when she was leaving for a few weeks to go to Finland to see her mother, I carefully arranged my injections to straddle her travel dates. On the visit prior to her departure, I knew I was getting two shots in the rear, so I had my husband write "bon voyage" with a marker across the injection site so she got a good laugh when I dropped my drawers!

And she's always surprising me too. I still have to look away while she's working, because I get queasy at

TEACHING MOMENT:

She always remembers whatever I tell her about my life and family, hopes and fears, and inquires about them at each visit.

the sight of blood, and I usually start humming something inane. Last week she chimed in, singing, in her native Finnish, a children's song about a pig that had me laughing so hard there were tears in my eyes. Tears of gratitude, for sure, because without Susanne I don't think I would have made it this far.

Susanne may not get as many nominations as other nurses in larger urban areas, but that doesn't mean she doesn't make an exponential difference with the patients that come her way. We live in a town of 10,000 after all, and have a small hospital. Astoria didn't even have a full-time oncologist until about a year ago. For me to be able to get this kind of care here, where I live, on a regular basis without having to travel, is extraordinarily helpful to me and healing in itself. She is my rock and helps me keep the faith that I can survive and thrive, no matter what the challenge. ❧

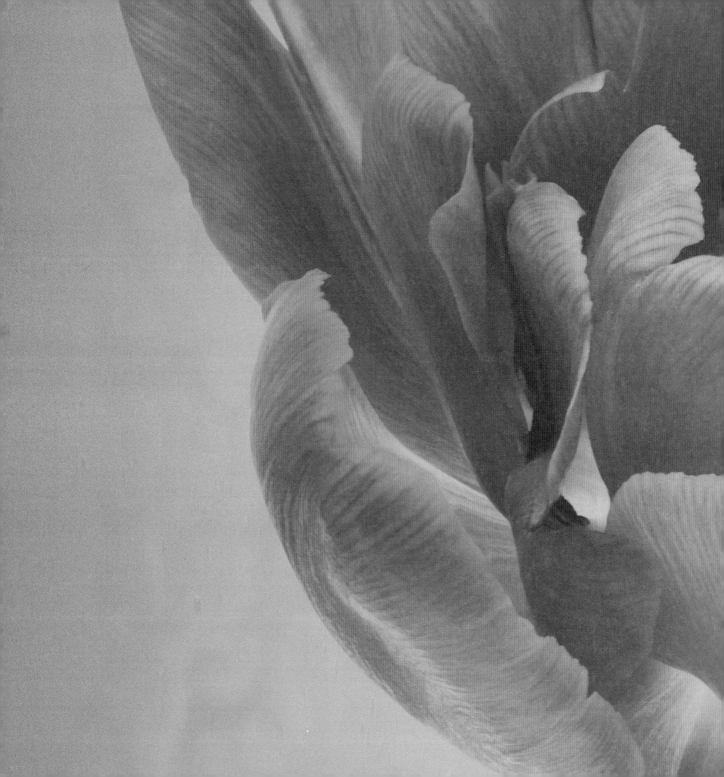

CHAPTER 5

Touching the Spirit

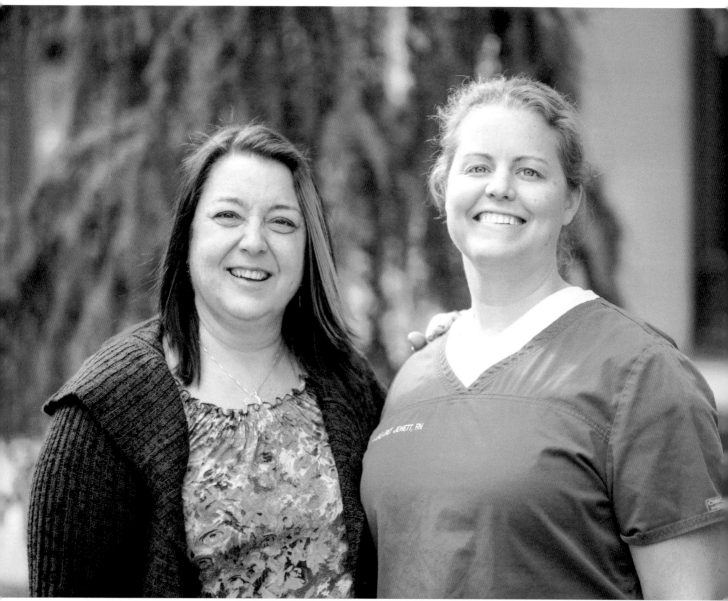

Susan Fariss with, Meg Jewett RN, BSN [right]

Hope in a Dark Place

MEG JEWETT, RN, BSN [KATZEN CANCER RESEARCH CENTER IN WASHINGTON, D.C.]

WRITTEN BY SUSAN FARISS

HOPE IS HARD TO FIND IN A CANCER WARD, especially when the news is stage 4 metastatic breast cancer to the liver. But hope is exactly what oncology nurse Meg Jewett has given me. I was diagnosed with stage 4 breast cancer from the get-go in February 2012. At first, my oncologist believed I was stage 2. My breast MRI showed no lymph node enlargement, and I was a young 47-year-old woman, so there was no reason to believe the cancer had spread. But a pre-treatment bone scan and CT scan showed otherwise. My liver was covered with lesions. As soon as I received the news, I began to split up my belongings in my head and plan my funeral.

IT WAS MEG WHO SAT DOWN NEXT TO ME, as I was receiving one of my first of 20 weekly paclitaxel infusions, and told me, "I know someone who is still alive 30 years later after a diagnosis of advanced cancer." And it has been Meg who has repeated that to me over and over again, as I've struggled to find hope in a dark and difficult situation.

Every week during my infusion, Meg met me with humor and a practical yet positive approach to cancer treatment. Meg was the one who instructed me on the vitamins to take to help alleviate my building neuropathy. It was Meg who reassured me that the side effects I was experiencing were normal and that I'd get through them. The lesions on my liver dropped to just scar tissue after five months of treatment, and I was stable on Herceptin for almost two years. When I finished the rounds of paclitaxel, I wanted to thank Meg by taking her out for a wonderful meal, but I had to settle for bringing food to her at the cancer center because she was too busy treating other patients.

In December 2013 the cancer came back, again to my liver. And again I dropped into hopelessness. Thankfully, Meg had previously talked about her experience during the clinical trials for Kadcyla, telling me how well the women on this drug did and how easily they tolerated it. With this progression, I was terrified to go through yet another round of knock-me-down chemo. Five months of weekly paclitaxel had almost disabled me and the resulting isolation sent me into a deep depression. As I was coming out of the examining room, after receiving the news of my progression, I saw Meg in the hallway. Wordlessly I walked over to her, hugged her and began to cry. Meg has become a steadying point, a buoy to grab onto in these very choppy cancerous seas. That hug gave me a glimmer that maybe things will be OK. I started Kadcyla two months ago.

I not only trust Meg's skills and knowledge as an oncology nurse, I trust her ability to always, always give me hope, even when things get really bad.

Hope. It's such a simple word, but yet so hard for many to give.

I not only trust Meg's skills and knowledge as an oncology nurse, I trust her ability to always, always give me hope, even when things get really bad. As Dr. Bernie Siegel puts it, medical staff can "deceive people into health" by simply treating them like they're going to live. And Meg has consistently treated me like I'm going to live. The best part is that Meg believes it herself. I can feel it; she believes I'm going to live. I don't care if either of us is deceiving ourselves. It matters. Words and actions matter.

Believing that I'm going to live keeps me going from day to day. And every three weeks I know I'll see Meg for my next dose of hope and Kadcyla. Meg has become a key member of my medical team, as important to me as my oncologist. And I am sure that Meg's continuing belief in my health has helped to keep me alive as surely as the chemotherapy has. ❧

Keeping Me Grounded to My Whole

AMY HARTMAN, RN, BSN, OCN [PROVIDENCE CANCER CENTER ONCOLOGY AND
HEMATOLOGY CARE CLINIC, EASTSIDE PORTLAND IN PORTLAND, OREGON]
WRITTEN BY KELLY SELIS

NURSES ARE DEFINITELY the unsung heroes of cancer treatment. They are on the frontline and can make the difference between just treatment and healing through treatment. When I first heard about nominating an oncology nurse for going above and beyond, I immediately thought of Amy Hartman.

AMY, ONE OF THE ONCOLOGY/HEMATOLOGY NURSES, went above and beyond for me just by being herself. I was diagnosed with breast cancer two years ago. My treatment after surgery was six rounds of chemo and a year of Herceptin.

It is hard on one's whole being to become a cancer patient. To face one's mortality, to lose one's hair, to feel like you somehow caused the cancer—all of these different aspects come crashing down on you as soon as you hear the word "cancer." And chemo is the added torture one has to deal with in addition to all the other aspects of cancer.

Plainly stated, going to chemotherapy sucks. No way around it—it sucks. My arm was poked, sometimes just once, sometimes several times, to start the IV. I almost passed out once from the pain and felt like a druggie with my bruised arm at times because I was adamant against getting a port. I felt awful for a few days after my treatment, as well as being exhausted most of the time. And the loss of hair does quite a job on one's self-esteem.

It came as quite a surprise when I found myself actually looking forward to going to chemo. Sounds pretty crazy, I know, and yet the reason was to see and talk to the nurses, mostly Amy. She helped make chemo day a tolerable day, one where I wasn't just a sick cancer patient, but a normal person having conversa-

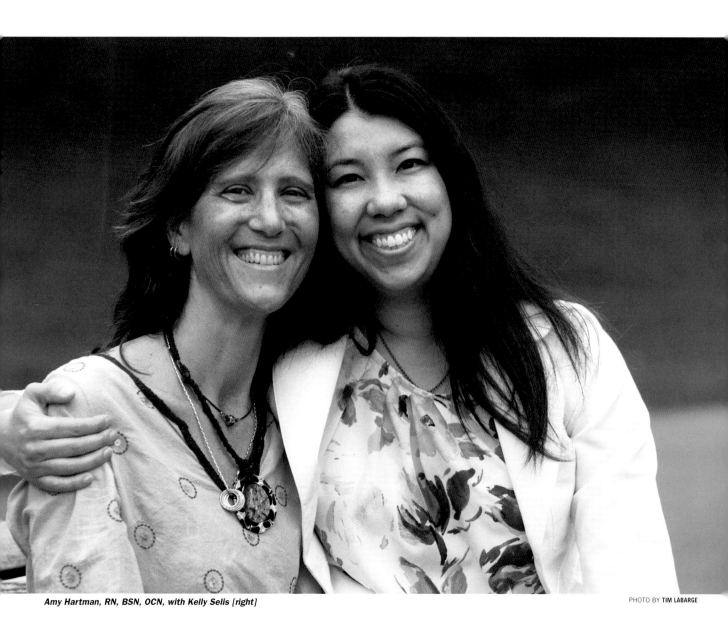

Amy Hartman, RN, BSN, OCN, with Kelly Selis [right]

tions about many different topics with her. She allowed me to stay connected to myself and not lose myself in the cancer patient role. When we talked, I felt heard by her and felt her genuine interest and concern in me, not just as a cancer patient, but as a whole person. She helped keep me grounded to who I am, to all of me, not just the cancer patient, which is how I often felt during that period.

She provided me with the little added touches to treatment that made all the difference, as well. The one time I almost fainted, she was so present with me, wiping my forehead with a warm washcloth and waiting until I had truly "returned" and the threat of fainting had passed. The time I had a severe, excruciating painful reaction to Emend was another example. Amy responded quickly to my husband's frantic cry for help, as I almost passed out from the pain. She was able to both calm my husband while also stopping the pain and dealing with the reaction quickly and professionally. Her soothing words and calm explanation of what was happening again helped keep me grounded at a very difficult time. And the time I called and left a cryptic message for her is yet another example. (I wasn't comfortable telling the operator why I was calling.) Amy immediately called back and spent a significant amount of time with me, answering my question and addressing, again, my whole being.

While I was in treatment, Amy went to Haiti with a medical group to do volunteer work. It was exciting to hear about the preparation, as well as the stories, when she returned. It also sparked a conversation about my own upcoming trip to Cuba to visit my father-in-law, a trip where planning also helped keep me going while in treatment. When she heard I was going, she graciously offered some of the leftover donations to take with me, which was quite a blessing.

In Cuba, I was able to give them to the head of oncology, who is a friend of a friend, at one of the hospitals. The Cuban doctor was thrilled to receive the donations, and again thanks to Amy, I had another opportunity to again not feel like a sick cancer patient, but a human connecting with others, helping others and not feeling so alone during my cancer journey.

Cancer sucks. Cancer treatment sucks, but with compassionate, caring medical providers, such as Amy, it becomes bearable. She made it not only bearable but allowed me to experience treatment, as I hope to experience all of life, as a whole person, connecting to others and feeling heard and understood. ✖

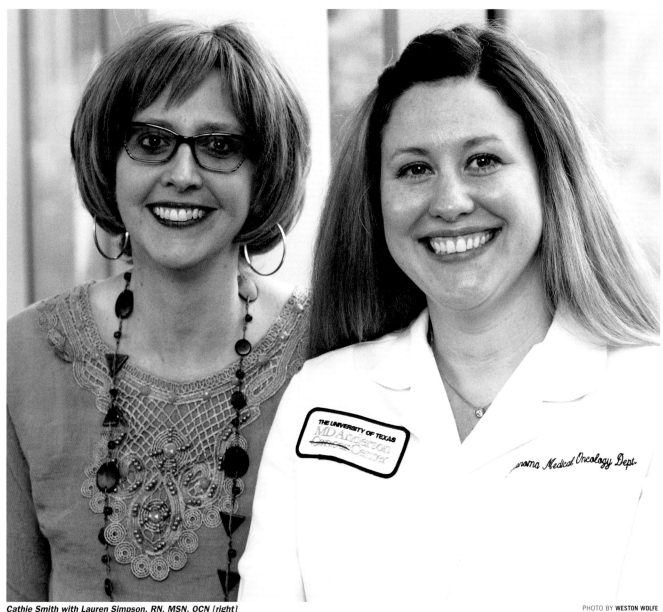

Cathie Smith with Lauren Simpson, RN, MSN, OCN [right]

Calm in the Storm

LAUREN SIMPSON, RN, MSN, OCN [MD ANDERSON CANCER CENTER IN HOUSTON, TEXAS]

WRITTEN BY CATHIE SMITH

MY HEART POUNDED as I awaited the news. I could hardly believe that my cancer had returned for a fourth time and this time was in my lungs. After multiple surgeries, various side effects and not being able to make any previous clinical trials, the news was devastating. I was now classified as having stage 4 melanoma and the prognosis was not good at all.

HOWEVER, FOR THE FIRST TIME, I finally qualified for a research trial. It would require many trips to my cancer center, and I would be assigned a research nurse that I was to be in close contact with at all times. That is where my calm in the storm comes into play.

Lauren Simpson, RN, melanoma and skin cancer research nurse, greeted me with a warm smile and patiently went over the many pages of details outlining the research study. She brought order to the seeming chaos and many details that seemed out of control. She was very positive and encouraging, and I was amazed at her wisdom and compassion well beyond her young age. After several appointments, I knew I had come upon a priceless treasure. She always entered the room with a beaming smile that could brighten even the darkest and most difficult days. You could sense the genuine compassion in her voice and her actions. She remembered almost every detail of my multiple side effects and symptoms and was on top of it with a plan every time. Again, she was able to calm the storm of side effects by coming up with yet another plan.

No matter how many times my husband or I had to call during the week, she greeted us with friendliness and warmth, and no question remained unanswered. If she did not know the answer right off, she immediately went to work to find it. I was in utter amazement of how tightly she worked with my oncologist and kept her up to speed on everything that was going on with me and worked to get me feeling better as soon as possible.

I had multiple side effects and many trips to the emergency room. Each time, she made me feel as if I were her very own family member and checked to see the progress I was making. She also went to find something to help me when expected progress was not taking place. She never seemed irritated or impatient, even with my multiple and seemingly never-ending questions. She was always very calming and reassuring. Some days, I even talked to her multiple times and she always received me with genuine friendliness and a listening ear. I always felt like I was talking to a dear friend, and for that alone she deserves a million accolades!

Even though she dealt with various patients, I was amazed at how she remembered each detail of my story, side effects and treatment plan. She never seemed rushed or bothered by the storms of side effects and patients she had around her. She was personally and emotionally committed and dedicated to my well being.

Lauren truly deserves recognition for her compassion, expertise and helpfulness. I have never met a nurse that was so on top of her game at such a very young age. She was always eager to help and to make me feel important and understood.

A cancer diagnosis is never easy, regardless of the stage. It truly feels like a storm that rages on and on without end. However, having caring and compassionate individuals like Lauren makes the healing process

TEACHING MOMENT:

She never seemed irritated or impatient, even with my multiple and seemingly never-ending questions. She was always very calming and reassuring.

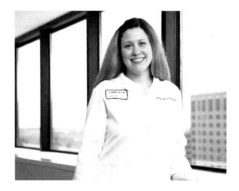

much smoother and gives the patient extra energy to fight the battle itself and not have to worry about the details.

I felt like I could focus on getting myself well and leave the details of the side effects and research in her hands. I knew she would keep me informed and would work as quickly as she could to work out problems and issues that came about in the process. I always felt like she understood me as an individual and she treated me like I was her only patient, even though she had several other patients each day.

Lauren Simpson, beyond a shadow of a doubt, deserves *CURE*'s 2014 Extraordinary Healer Award for Oncology Nursing for helping to be the calm in my cancer storm. She exudes genuine compassion, amazing knowledge and expertise, around-the-clock helpfulness and amazing attention to detail. I will forever be grateful for Lauren for being in my life and being such an important part of my healing process. My storm is not over, but I am thankful that Lauren is a part of the calm in the storm. ✖

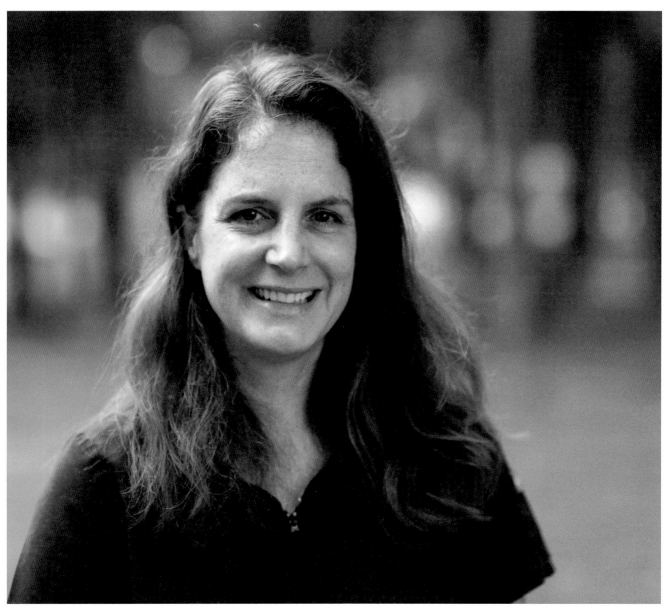

Regina "Gina" Ayers, RN, OCN

The Extraordinary Everyday Healer

REGINA "GINA" AYERS, RN, OCN [FLORIDA CANCER AFFILIATES IN LADY LAKE, FLORIDA]

WRITTEN BY DIANE BRANDLEY

SOME CANCER TREATMENT CENTERS are mere conveyer belts for infusion. Then there are those that transform the experience into a time of caring and spiritual healing. In a small satellite office of a large oncology practice, one nurse—the only nurse—makes that happen.

EARLY IN 2012, my husband Ted's care was transferred to Ocala Oncology, now a part of Florida Cancer Affiliates, in Ocala, Florida. He has been dealing with prostate cancer for 14 years and started on a new state-of-the-art treatment. Our hopes were high that this medication would be the answer—not a cure, but at least a period of remission. Unexpectedly, in May of that year, I became a patient as well after being diagnosed with ovarian cancer.

During the initial visit, my heart fell. The satellite center is a cheerless, windowless place. We met Regina Ayers, the oncology nurse who directs treatment for all of the patients. Her manner assured us that the cheer and the light came from within the spirit of the four-person team and the bonds that formed among patients. While treatment held its difficulties, it turned out she was right about spirit and bonds.

Like most infusion centers, the action is nonstop. Seven reclining chairs serve a continuing stream of patients. Alarms punctuate the calm, many of them sounding at the same time. The challenge is managing situations that arise suddenly. Equipment malfunctions. Patients develop complications. Drugs must be given in sequence. Physicians require unique responses to their particular management styles. Some cancer patients are scared, some are angry, some of us just want to be rid of our burden of treatment and act out accordingly.

These issues are a fact of life which Gina describes as "trying to put together a puzzle. Nothing is more stressful than boredom and nothing more satisfying than being relevant and privileged enough to make a difference."

For her, the puzzles are endless. She addresses malfunctions with persistence, competing alarms with unflappable patience. Patient complications are always the priority, yet they take their place in the queue of priorities, always in collaboration with respective physicians. One day, I witnessed a couple arguing, making no effort to hide their hostility from any of us. The patient was about to be hospitalized directly from the center. While Gina made every effort to support them during the transfer, she later conveyed her understanding about their anger, feeling that much of it was covering fear.

Gina developed compassion from two sources. The first was family. She is one of four natural and three adopted siblings. There were countless foster children in and out of the household. Gina and her husband have two children from the foster care system as well. Her mother worked as a nursing assistant throughout her career. In sharing anecdotes from work, her mother conveyed the importance of the relationship with patients, even those who were not conscious. She saw the effect of a comatose patient change completely when a nurse referred to her as having a "wasted life"—a lesson not lost on Gina.

The second source was her personal health experiences. At age 12, doctors suspected leukemia. This revelation was terrifying, but eventually proved to be incorrect. Numerous surgeries and the loss of a baby have strengthened her resolve to be helpful to other people during their time of need. After making her way up the career ladder from vocational nurse to registered nurse, she aspired to become an oncology nurse.

Throughout treatment, I personally felt that when my turn came for attention, I was the only patient in the room. From visit to visit, she remembered the books I was reading and shared information about the books on tape that she played for her kids en route to school and activities. We often shared travel and family information. While her mind constantly monitored the treatment plans for seven patients, her attention was fixed; the patient in front of her was the only focus.

As my chemotherapy treatments ended, Ted's was just beginning. We joked that I had warmed a chair for him, but humor aside, we were devastated. For him, it's a literal roulette game of treatment and the options are running out.

Gina is "there" for him at every turn, and in so doing, reminds me of a quote from another nurse's memoir: "I learned that many times there was nothing to say, that sometimes just not turning away from people was the best way to care for them," *Beautiful Unbroken: One Nurse's Life* by Mary Jane Nealon

There are so many nurses quietly working day to day whose skills and quiet compassion provide either the spiritual healing or peaceful acceptance so necessary for a patient. Gina provides both for us. We continue our course of treatment and follow-up, along with a determination to live our days by squeezing the marrow out of each one, and never giving up.

We are so much the richer for having her in our lives. ❧

TEACHING MOMENT:

While her mind constantly monitored the treatment plans for seven patients, her attention was fixed; the patient in front of her was the only focus.

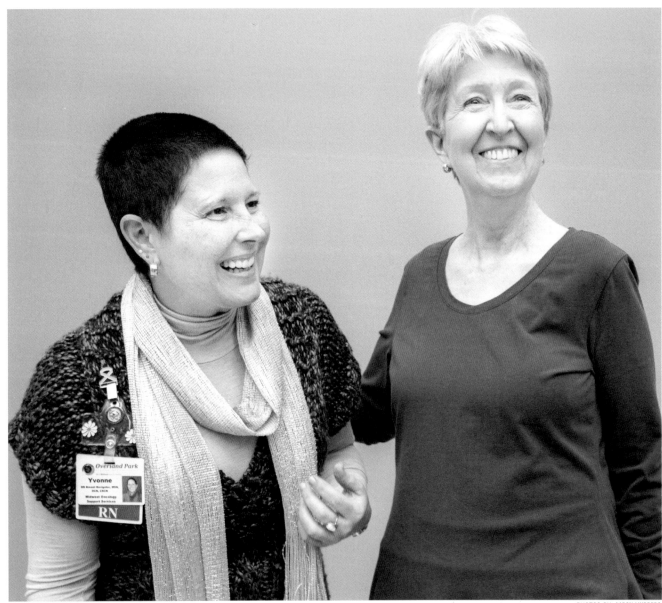

Yvonne Ward, RN, BSN, OCN, with Rose Niland [right]

The Card of Hope, The Card of Life

YVONNE WARD, RN, BSN, OCN, CBCN

[THE UNIVERSITY OF KANSAS CANCER CENTER IN WESTWOOD, KANSAS]

WRITTEN BY ROSE NILAND

LONG AFTER THE TREATMENT ENDED, the card lived. It lived in my purse, in my Rolodex file and in my kitchen drawer. That little flexible piece of cardboard was more powerful than a credit card, driver's license or lottery ticket and held such comfort, such reassurance, such hope. That card was the link to my caring nurse, Yvonne Ward.

MY TREATMENT JOURNEY started on a hot day in July 2011 at the breast cancer clinic at the University of Kansas Cancer Center in a nondescript conference room. Nothing stood out in that room to distract me. My bewildered husband was at my side. I had little to stare at but the truth through the eyes of Dr. Sharma, my oncologist. I listened, but only two words stood out during that frank consultation, with "aggressive" being the first word describing my stage 3 ductal carcinoma.

I was shocked. At no time in my 58 years of life had I ever been aggressive in any way until now. I was nonconfrontational by nature, but now I had an aggressive component—and it was cancer. The details droned on with unfamiliar acronyms like HER2, ER and PR, sounding in my numbed brain like an alphabet soup of terms and symbols. I felt how an animal must feel when listening to humans talk. It was a lot of "blah, blah, blah" until an occasional familiar word jumped out like "outside, walk or treat." Suddenly the second word jumped out: curable. In fact, she said "100 percent curable."

What? How could that be? After all, I have stage 3 aggressive breast cancer. Did I hear her correctly? In my brain, the negativity of the term "aggressive" was battling with the hope of "100 percent curable." I had a lot to think about.

The next step was to finalize my chemotherapy schedule, and that's when I got "the card" and Yvonne Ward entered my life. When I first saw her I was intrigued, yet curious. She had a big smile, a shaved head and a bag holding a big red notebook. Why was her head shaved? How could she be so cheerful when she had to deal with cancer patients every day? What is in that oversized notebook?

Bewildered and apprehensive, we followed Yvonne through the maze of cubicles within the massive treatment area while she explained the procedures and showed us one of the cubicles that would be my private haven for several hours at a time. We visited the lounge and snack area. She even demonstrated how I could walk to the restroom with all of my paraphernalia traveling along for the ride. So I thought, "Now, I guess I'm ready."

But there was more. Yvonne was by my side, showing me the notebook. Now, I would find out the mystery of the red notebook. It was my personal treatment plan, including lists of possible concerns, side effects of the particular chemo cocktail I was receiving and a reputable website I could visit for more information, suggested foods to eat and strategies to make my life more comfortable. The notebook was my bible of hope, and her business card was my lifeline with the phone number I could call with questions, concerns observations or reminders. She made me feel I could call her even when I wasn't sure if I should. The card was just as important to me as the fleece blanket that kept me warm as I lay in the recliner at home on the days following a treatment session. The card followed me to appointments, to work and to infrequent coffee dates with friends.

Chemo counseling was my first positive experience in this treatment journey. Yvonne made no promises. She was a superb caring professional in every way. She was upbeat and personable. She accepted my crying fits as I stared at the number of chemo rooms and the volume of patients being treated, and later as I examined my lab numbers that ultimately delayed my scheduled treatment and required another unit of blood instead. She made appointments when I was in a panic about an eye infection, gave suggestions to identify the cause of a rash and was a liaison to Dr. Sharma when my anti-nausea meds weren't helping like I thought they should. She made sure I had signatures and all of the information I needed to file cancer insurance claims.

Some might say she was just doing her job. True, but it was much more than that. Others might say a nurse coordinator couldn't get close enough to make a profound difference in a cancer patient's life. I disagree.

I had many caring chemo nurses, but each treatment brought yet another smiling nurse. Unlike Yvonne, there was no consistency. I found myself looking for her at every oncology appointment. She remembered us. She followed our journey. She noticed when my hair grew back in an unexpected shade of grey. She cared. I wanted to make her proud as I continued to be a compliant patient and did my part in my yearlong treatment plan. Besides my husband, she was the most positive and predictable factor in my unpredictable road to survival.

Although my treatment has ended, I continue to look for Yvonne at my six-month checkups. I keep track of the glimmer of her smile, that same caring voice and upbeat attitude with the new patients and the length of her hair. Oh yes, she originally shaved her head for a charity cause and continues to keep it closely cropped! She's still there for me—for all of us.

The three copies of "the card" are still with me. I am staring at the one from my Rolodex as I write this tribute. Yes, it's only a calling card, but it was also my confidence, my crutch, my hope, my friend on a piece of cardstock: Yvonne Ward, RN, BSN, OCN, CBCN, my truly extraordinary caring nurse. ❧

TEACHING MOMENT:

I wanted to make her proud as I continued to be a compliant patient and did my part in my yearlong treatment plan. Besides my husband, she was the most positive and predictable factor in my unpredictable road to survival.

My Angel Nurse

AMBER JACKSON, RN, BSN, OCN

[SUSAN P. WHEATLAKE REGIONAL CANCER CENTER IN REED CITY, MISSOURI]

WRITTEN BY EMILY PONTZ

IT IS IN THE DARKEST of moments of one's life that the light is truly able to shine through. That light can come in many forms. Mine came in the form of my chemo nurse, Amber, whom I also lovingly call, Angel Nurse.

I WAS RECENTLY DIAGNOSED with a very aggressive form of breast cancer. Breast cancer is no stranger to women of all backgrounds. It usually chooses its victims regardless of many factors. I, however, am 24 years old. With all of my life in front of me, a fear began to take hold. Would I live to see the day I would marry the love of my life? Would I ever hold my baby in my arms? I was confronted with many questions such as these and had only my faith to guide me forward.

Walking into my first day of chemotherapy, I was both scared and ready; scared for the effects it may have on my ability to have children and ready to kill any remaining cancer that may be harboring itself in my body. And then I met Amber and my fears subsided until all that was left was strength and perseverance.

Amber has the two things that make a good nurse a great one, one that changes lives. She is so proficient and dedicated to her work that she makes one of the most horrific experiences (chemotherapy) absolutely bearable. This proficiency was just rewarded as she was appointed the nurse in charge of infusion therapy at the Susan P. Wheatlake Cancer Center. Secondly, and more importantly, she heals with her ability to care for her patients on a personal level. I learned how truly crucial this aspect of treatment is when my father, who recently received a heart transplant, was ill for many years, and again when my mother died suddenly only months later. The nurses that care for their patients on a personal level make such a difference that it is immeasurable.

I continued on with my treatments, and I understood fully that when people spoke of their "battle" with cancer, they were referring to the emotional and mental battle even more than the physical one. Amber helped to heal me physically, but her hand in healing me mentally and emotionally will last until the day I leave this earth. Her constant smile reminded me that there is beauty and friendship that can be found in the struggle. Above all, she made me feel safe. She allowed me the ability to see and plan for my future.

On one of my many rough days during chemotherapy, I lost consciousness during my appointment with my oncologist. I awoke to countless people surrounding me and could feel tears streaming down my face as I lay there. It was one of the scariest moments of my life thus far. And then Amber stood above me and told me it would all be OK and that she would never let anything happen to me. She wiped the tears from my face and kissed my forehead. Seeing her and knowing she was there erased any fears I may have had.

She truly was and will forever be my Angel Nurse. I credit her with saving my life in more ways than one. As I write this, I cannot help but to cry and smile all at once. My words cannot begin to describe this wonderful person, but I knew when I saw *CURE*'s question, "Do you know an extraordinary oncology nurse?" I had to write you and say, "Yes! I know the very best one!" ❧

TEACHING MOMENT:

Amber helped to heal me physically,
but her hand in healing me mentally
and emotionally will last until the day
I leave this earth.

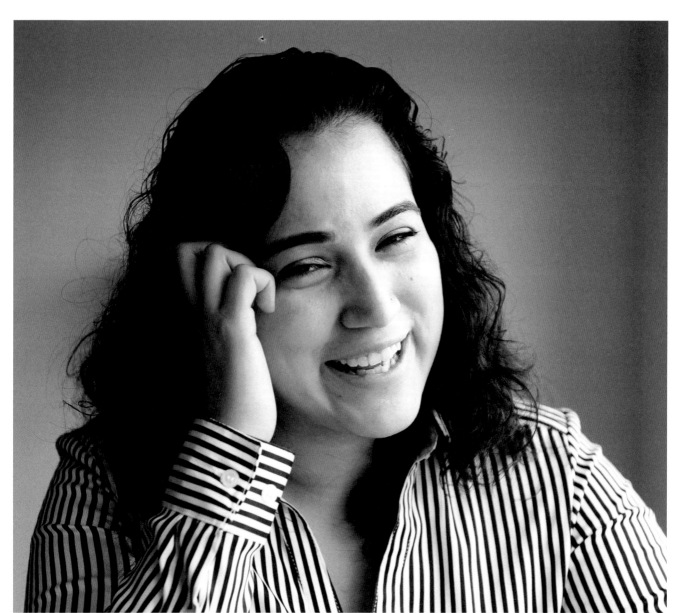

Yesenia Nunez, RN, BSN

An Exceptional Healer in MyelomaLand

YESENIA NUNEZ, RN, BSN

[UNIVERSITY OF MARYLAND MARLENE AND STEWART GREENEBAUM CANCER CENTER IN BALTIMORE, MARYLAND]

WRITTEN BY STEPHEN EISENBERG

IT IS WITH ENTHUSIASM that I nominate Yesenia Nunez, RN, for *CURE*'s 2014 Extraordinary Healer Award for Oncology Nursing. While I consider the entire nursing staff of the Blood and Marrow Transplant Unit of the University of Maryland Greenbaum Cancer Center to be excellent, Ms. Nunez is exceptional.

MS. NUNEZ RECEIVED HER BACHELOR OF SCIENCE in nursing from the Catholic University of America in Washington, D.C., in 2011, and became a registered nurse in August 2011. She was certified in chemotherapy and biotherapy administration through the University of Maryland Medical School in February 2012.

This is where I had the good fortune to meet Ms. Nunez. I am a 62-year-old dentist who was diagnosed with multiple myeloma two years ago. I received an autologous stem cell transplant in October 2013. Due to a relapse of the myeloma, I was re-hospitalized in January 2014 for chemotherapy and a reintroduction of my stem cells.

Ms. Nunez was my primary nurse for both admissions. Over my five weeks of hospitalizations, Ms. Nunez was a consistent source of empathy and concern for my comfort and well-being. She was also my conduit to positive thinking, which is essential for recovery.

My experience as a health care professional is in dealing with the many physical and psychological needs of relatively healthy people on an outpatient basis. The Blood and Marrow Transplant Unit is a far different world, as the patients are in debilitative physical and emotional states in a restrictive hospital unit. It takes a special person to work on a daily basis with this patient population. Ms. Nunez is that special person.

Aside from her excellent nursing skills, she made herself available to answer questions about my progress. Without using medical jargon, Ms. Nunez often explained my treatment to my family and how I was progressing in my journey through "Myelomaland." She also very clearly explained to my family how to handle the restrictions I would be under at home. Her manner was very nonthreatening and sometimes humorous. Ms. Nunez was a source of comfort to me and my family.

I was despondent eight weeks after my first discharge when I learned I had to return to the unit, as my stem cell transplant failed. Yet, although this quick return was not on my bucket list, the calm and kind manner in which Ms. Nunez welcomed me and eased my transition back into the unit helped me to quickly adjust once again to the routine of being a hospitalized cancer patient. While not exactly a welcome homecoming, I was quickly put at ease emotionally, my depression subsided and I felt that the unit was my home away from home.

One of Ms. Nunez's great interpersonal skills is engaging in topics of interest to the patient while fulfilling her nursing duties. Ms. Nunez facilitated countless impromptu medical and dental discussions with me. While I read as much as I can on multiple myeloma, there is a disconnect between scientific papers and the actual treatment modalities. Ms. Nunez helped bridge that knowledge gap in explaining why my physician wanted to do procedure A instead of B at a certain point in time. In return, I explained basic dentistry and proper oral hygiene, most important for cancer patients. I hope I was able to impart some of my knowledge to the Blood and Marrow Transplant Unit staff and improve the survival rate of their patients.

Ms. Nunez gave me the sense that I was of help to the unit in answering questions about dental conditions that compromise cancer treatments. In doing so, she helped me believe that I remained essential and still had worth, despite my cancer.

I see Ms. Nunez as the quintessential oncology nurse, who is hands-on, knowledgeable and compassionate. The likelihood is that I will need another stem cell transplant. Being a regular on the unit is not as daunting a thought knowing I will be under the care of Ms. Nunez or one her excellent colleagues. ❧

2014 Extraordinary Healer Award for Oncology Nursing

Nominees

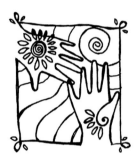

CURE congratulates each nurse who was nominated. You are all extraordinary healers.

Kathy Ammirata / Florida Cancer Care

Michele Anderson / Compass Oncology

Molly Antony / Detroit Medical Center Huron Valley-Sinai Hospital

Jeannine Arias / Adventist Hinsdale Hospital
and Adventist La Grange Memorial Hospital

Calvin Askew / Northside Hospital Cancer Institute

Regina Ayers / Florida Cancer Affiliates

Leslie Bainbridge / Arizona Oncology

Loretta Balentine / Midwest Cancer Care Belton Regional Medical Center

Eileen Bannon / Penn State Hershey Medical Center

Shonnette Bennett / Florida Hospital Memorial
Medical Center Cancer Institute

Susanne Benthin / Columbia Memorial Hospital

Charlene Brady / Metcare Oncology

Jackie Broadway-Duren / MD Anderson Cancer Center

Ann Bunyan / New York Oncology Hematology

Angela Caballero / The Cancer Centers at Saint Barnabas Medical Center

Joanne Candela / Memorial Sloan Kettering Cancer Center

Cindi Cantril / Sutter Pacific Medical Foundation

Elizabeth "Beth" Casey / St. Jude Children's Research Hospital

Mary Chacko / MD Anderson Cancer Center

Stephanie Clapham / Mercy Health Saint Mary's

Diane Cope / Florida Cancer Specialists and Research Institute

Linda Cox / St. Luke's Mountain States Tumor Institute

Danielle Dambro / Chester County Hospital

Chanda Danczak / California Cancer Associates for Research & Excellence

Jan Day / Texas Oncology

Saskia de Koomen / The Huntington Hospital Cancer Center

Leta Deskins Rex / Hematology Oncology Associates

Rosalee Di Salvo Rethoret / Carl T. Hayden Veterans Affairs
Medical Center

Mary Dibley / James P. Wilmot Cancer Center, University of
Rochester Medical Center

Jennifer Donahue / Florida Hospital
Memorial Medical Center Cancer Institute

Deborah Doss / Dana-Farber Cancer Institute

Lenora Drum / Office of Dr. Neelesh S. Bangalore

Arlene Dyer / NorthShore University HealthSystem

Mary Jane Fahrenkrug / Seattle Cancer Care Alliance

Pamela Falco / Florida Hospital
Memorial Medical Center Cancer Institute

Dana Ferrence / Florida Hospital
Memorial Medical Center Cancer Institute

Judy Gardiner / Paragon Healthcare

Susan "Sue" Gentry / Texas Oncology

Teresa Gonzalez / Kaiser Permanente,
South Bay Medical Center

Ann Grotz / Compass Oncology

Irene Haapoja / Rush University Medical Center

Diana Hahn / Compass Oncology

Sue Hamilton / Texas Oncology

Nancy Hampton-Jones / Mercy Health

Theresa Hanlin / Sentara Virgina Beach General Hospital

Michael Hargens / Marshfield Clinic

Joanne Harkness / Johns Hopkins Hospital

Jeanie Harris / Florida Cancer Specialists & Research Institute

Amy Hartman / Providence Cancer Center Oncology and
Hematology Care Clinic

Megan Haun / Gundersen Health System

Allison Haynes-Johnson / Arizona Oncology

Nancy Heather / Contra Costa Oncology

Verna Hendricks-Ferguson / Saint Louis University
School of Nursing

Brittany Hendrix / University of Mississippi Medical Center

Lucy Hertel / Barnes-Jewish Hospital,
Division of Gynecologic Oncology

Patti Higginbotham / Alegent Creighton Breast
Health Center - Lakeside

Robin Hinckley / MultiCare Regional Cancer Center

Kim Hinnebusch / Halvorson Cancer Center

Karyn Hoikka / University of Minnesota
Medical Center, Fairview

Delores "Maxine" Howard / Northwest Alabama
Cancer Center

Amanda Hughes / Memorial Sloan Kettering Cancer Center

Thelma Hulka / Adventist Hinsdale Hospital

Amber Jackson / Susan P. Wheatlake
Regional Cancer Center

Margaret "Meg" Jewett / The Katzen Cancer Research Center at
The George Washington University

Linda Joice / Compass Oncology

Beverly Kidd / William Beaumont Army Medical Center

Barbara Kingsbury / Orange Coast Memorial Medical Center

Susan Kinnear Segreti / VA Health Care of Upstate New York

Paula LaBarge / Dutchess Hematology Oncology

Maureen Laffey / Memorial Sloan Kettering Cancer Center

Kathleen Larson / Memorial Sloan Kettering Cancer Center

Debra Anne Lawry / AMGEN Oncology

Colleen Lewis / Winship Cancer Institute of Emory University

Wendy Lien / SkyRidge Medical Center

Claudia Lopez / Texas Oncology

Jenny Lott / Northwestern Medical Faculty Foundation

Mary Bess Luitwieler / Hematology Oncology Consultants

Kristy Maida-LaMere / Memorial Sloan Kettering Cancer Center

Kathleen Maignan / Columbia Doctors Midtown,
Columbia University Medical Center

Gretchen Marino / Memorial Sloan Kettering Cancer Center

Anne Markham / Thomas Jefferson University

Debra Mascarenhas / Vidant Medical Center

Cynthia "Cindy" May / Greater Houston Cancer Clinic

Martha May / St. Jude Children's Research Hospital

Betty McEver / Cayuga Medical Center

Cara McKellar / Community Howard Regional Health

Mary Milar / Florida Hospital
Memorial Medical Center Cancer Institute

Theresa "Terry" Minieri / Medical Specialists of the Palm Beaches

Linda Mitchell / Porter Cancer Care Center

Treasa Mooney / Eastern Maine Medical Center Cancer Care of Maine

Alida Moore / Spectrum Health Medical Group

Iva Morris / Charles George VA Medical Center

Nancy Mortlock / Evergreen Hematology and Oncology

Cheryl Muldoon / UF Health Cancer Center at Orlando Health

Pat Nockels / Medical Oncology and Hematology Associates at
John Stoddard Cancer Center

Denise Norfolk / Florida Hospital
Memorial Medical Center Cancer Institute

Yesenia Nunez / University of Maryland Greenebaum Cancer Center

Patricia "Pat" O'Nan / Florida Hospital
Memorial Medical Center Cancer Institute

Charlene Parker / Kaiser Permanente - Oncology Department

Noelle Paul / Memorial Sloan Kettering Cancer Center

Barbara Peters / Intermountain Health Care
Janice Beesley Hartvigsen Breast Care Center

Lisa Pope / Vita Medical Associates

Veronica Ramirez / San Antonio Community Hospital

Macey Reeves-Alexander / UT Southwestern,
Harold C. Simmons Cancer Center

Carol Rhoades / Cancer Care Centers of South Texas

Kathie Jo Ritchey / Virginia K. Crosson Cancer Center

Melinda Roach / Virginia Commonwealth University

Massey Cancer Center

Amy Roudebush / Midwest Cancer Care Belton

Regional Medical Center

Sarah Rowe / Pan Coastal Hematology Oncology

Lauren Simpson / MD Anderson Cancer Center

Stephanie Smith / Midwest Cancer Care Belton

Regional Medical Center

Natalie Snyder / University of Minnesota

Amplatz Children's Hospital

Danielle Stanley / Vanderbilt-Ingram Cancer Center

Jennifer Stevick / Williamson Medical Center

Robin Swearingin / Exempla Lutheran Medical Center

Comprehensive Cancer Center

Teri Tasler / Duke Raleigh Cancer Center

Sandra "Sandy" Terrazzino / San Antonio

Military Medical Center

Megan Thacker / University of Maryland, Upper Chesapeake

Medical Center Kaufman Cancer Center

Kristen Thompson / Kapiolani Medical Center

for Women & Children

Cindy Thorton / Florida Hospital

Memorial Medical Center Cancer Institute

Anne Todd / Southern Indiana Physicans IU Health Oncology

Leigh Turner / Midwest Cancer Care Belton

Regional Medical Center

Lori Tuttle / Bay State Regional Cancer Program Pierre Valentini

Comprehensive Cancer Centers of Nevada

Janell Verkaden / Florida Hospital

Memorial Medical Center Cancer Institute

Barbara Wagner Dandorph / Indian Hill School, Holmdel

Township Public Schools

Suzanne Walker / Abramson Cancer Center of

the University of Pennsylvania

Yvonne Ward / Overland Park Regional Medical Center

Margaret Whalen / NorthShore University HealthSystem

Katina Wilson / Florida Hospital Celebration Health

Laura Wood / Cleveland Clinic Taussig Cancer Institute

Amy Youman / Florida Hospital

Memorial Medical Center Cancer Institute

Mary Beth Zill / Adventist La Grange Memorial Hospital